Introduction

On Tuesday November 25, 2015, the Department of Health and Human Service and CMS (Center for Medicare and Medicaid Services) produced its "Final Rule" for Comprehensive Care for Joint Replacement Payment Model for Acute Care Hospitals Furnishing Lower Extremity Joint Replacement Services; Final Rule. We will refer to this as CJR.[1] We also refer to this as bundled payment. For a few years before this ruling, there were experimental, voluntary government projects assessing the feasibility of doing this type of project. The early program was called BPCI (Bundled Payments for Care Improvement). There are two very important distinctions between BPCI and CJR. First, BPCI was voluntary and CJR is required. The second is that various groups such as Independent Practitioner Associations were able to take risk in BPCI but in CJR, only hospitals are able to do this.

This manual summarizes the 282-page ruling in a readable form. Keep in mind that this book was written to give the Orthopaedic community a chance to get through the entire ruling in a reasonable amount of time. We do not assure complete accuracy or interpretation of the actual ruling and cannot be held accountable by any actions you take by reading this book. This is for educational purposes only. You are encouraged to seek professional consultative and legal advice when embarking on CJR.

Let's get started.

Ira H. Kirschenbaum, MD
Chairman, Department of Orthopaedic Surgery
Bronx-Lebanon Hospital Center
Bronx, NY

---

[1] As an interesting note- it originally was CCJR but the US Government was sent a cease and desist letter from a registered trademark CCJR that stood for Current Concepts in Joint Replacement.

The Big Summary

In 2014 CMS paid claims on over 430,000 joint replacement cases. To increase coordination of care, maintain or improve outcomes, and optimize utilization, in 67 regions, called MSA's, all lower extremity joint replacement (LEJR) admissions (MS-DRG 469 and MS-DRG-470) to acute care hospitals will be required to be part of the CJR program. CMS will continue paying hospitals and other providers and suppliers according to the usual Medicare Fee-for-Service (FFS) payment systems during all performance years (5 years). After the completion of a performance year, the Medicare claims payments for services furnished to the beneficiary during the episode, based on claims data, will be combined to calculate an actual episode payment. The actual episode payment is the sum of Medicare Part A and B claims payments for all related items and services furnished to a beneficiary during a CJR episode. The actual episode payment will then be reconciled against an established CJR target price, with consideration of additional payment adjustments based on quality performance and post episode spending. The amount of this calculation, if positive, will be paid to the participant hospital (that may have collaborators with risk-sharing relationships) if the hospital has met the quality thresholds finalized in this rule. This payment is the reconciliation payment. If negative, the participant hospital (and collaborators) will be required to make repayment to Medicare. CMS is phasing in the requirement that hospitals whose actual episode payments exceed their CJR target price will need to pay the difference back to Medicare beginning in performance year 2. Medicare will not require repayment from hospitals for CJR episode spending above their target price in performance year 1. Lastly, CMS decided to limit how much a hospital can gain or lose based on its reconciliation calculation with additional policies to further limit the risk of high payment cases for all participant hospitals and for special categories of hospitals.

What is CJR?

Comprehensive Care in Joint Replacement (CJR) is a payment system to promote quality and financial responsibility in Lower Extremity Joint Replacement (LEJR)

CJR details are posted on the CMS website:
http://innovation.cms.gov/initiatives/cjr/

This link has the following important files:

- Press Release
- Consumer Fact Sheet (PDF)
- Provider and Technical Fact Sheet (PDF)
- Frequently Asked Questions (PDF)
- MSA volume and inclusion criteria worksheet (XLS)
- MSAs by population and payments (XLS)
- Hospital List (XLS)
- Episode exclusions (XLS)
- Average Regional Historical Episodes from Proposed Rule (XLS)
- ICD-9 and ICD-10 Hip Fracture Diagnosis Codes (XLS)
- Quality Strategy Supplemental Information (PDF)

CJR is under the authority of the Center for Medicare and Medicaid Innovation (CMMI).

Through CJR, CMS wants to reduce spending while maintain or improving quality. It covers inpatient and post-acute care (PAC).

This is a limited time test- April 1, 2016- December 31, 2020.

Payments are designed to stimulate infrastructure building. Medicare expects that hospitals will reinvest in the program to gain more efficiencies.

The acute care hospital that is the site of surgery is held accountable.

There is an opportunity for performance-based payments by reducing expenses and meeting quality metrics.

The role of physicians in this model, especially physicians who enter into sharing arrangement with CJR hospitals, is currently not fully worked out. The significance is whether this combination of CJR and shared arrangement would qualify as an alternate payment model (APM) having physicians qualify under the Medicare

Access and Chip Reauthorization Act of 2015. A further ruling will come out later but this has no bearing at this time on the current CJR rules.

Under the current Inpatient Prospective Payment System (IPPS), Lower Extremity Joint Replacement (LEJR) is covered through MS-DRG 469 (LEJR with major complication or comorbidity) and MS-DRG470 (LEJR without major comorbidity or complication). These are the only two MS-DRGs covered in CJR

The payment starts 3 days prior to admission and ends 90 days after discharge.

Payments include all Part A and Part B payments.

Only participating hospitals are the episode initiators and bear financial responsibility. ACOs, Medical Homes, and other conveners cannot initiate or administrate an episode.

All hospitals, within specific geographic regions determined by CMS that are currently paid under IPPS will be required to participate in CJR. As such, these hospitals are participating hospitals.

Eligible beneficiaries (patients) admitted to these hospitals are automatically enrolled.

The actual episode payments are calculated at the end of a performance year, based on claims data. These are reconciled against an established CJR target price.

Additional payment adjustments will be made based on quality performance, post-episode spending, and policies to limit hospital financial responsibility.

If the amount of difference between the CJR target and the actual payments is positive, then the hospital will be eligible for an additional payment from CMS. If that difference is negative, the hospital will have to repay a certain amount back to CMS based on the composite quality score

In Year 1 of the program there will be no reconciliation payments or repayments. All reconciliation payments and repayments will start in Year 2 and continue throughout the entire 5 years of the program.

There is a limit, though, to how much hospitals can actually gain or lose in subsequent years.

Certain hospitals that have been participating in risk-bearing phases BPCI 2 and 4 are being excluded from CJR as well as acute care hospitals participating in BPCI 1

Quality measures and reporting requirements include a complications measure and a patient experience survey measure. The scores will be posted on *Hospital*

Compare Web Site.

There is also voluntary submission of data related to Patient-Reported Outcomes.

Summary data between participating hospitals will be coordinated by CMMI.

CMMI will provide hospitals with up to 3 years of claims data that will be used to develop their target price.

Patients have the right to seek care during the CJR program with any qualified CMS provider. If the surgery is done at a CJR hospital, then the payment model is triggered and the patient can't opt out of the model.

Participating hospitals have to provide written information to patients about the program and patients' rights under the program.

CMMI reserves the right to audit hospitals to investigate inappropriate changes in delivered services.

Participating hospitals are required to assure that other providers and services collaborating with them agree to the terms of the model including all applicable program policy waivers.

There are certain conditions in which Skilled Nursing Facilities (SNFs) and physicians can bill the participating hospital for services not normally covered by Medicare.

The Secretary of HHS can terminate this entire program if it does not meet the economic and quality projections it has made.

The bundled payment will be paid retrospectively through a reconciliation process.

All CMS providers will continue to submit claims and receive payments via the usual Medicare FFS payment systems.

Provisions of the Proposed Regulations

The episode that triggers entry into the bundle is admission to an acute care hospital.

Hospitals are the only episode initiators in CJR. Hospitals in Maryland are excluded because that state entered into an agreement with CMS called the Maryland All-Payer Model.

In the voluntary BPCI Model 2 bundled payment system, health systems, physician-hospital organizations, physician group practices (PGPs), and non-provider business entities that act as conveners initiated episodes of care. In CJR, only hospitals can initiate an episode.

Many commenters to this Final Rule argued against only hospitals as CJR initiators but the issue is closed. Non-acute care hospital conveners are not initiators.

HHVBP (Home Health Value Based Purchasing) participants are not exempt from CJR.

ACOs are not exempt from CJR.

HRRP (Hospital Readmissions Reduction Program) participants are not exempt from CJR.

For hospitals that share a CCN (CMS Certification Number), all hospitals would be required to participate in CJR. The requirement for participation is the physical address of the hospital on the CCN and whether it is in the geographic area of the CJR program.

Participation in CJR has no LEJR case volume requirements. CMS did this to prevent shifting of higher cost cases to other institutions

Regions were determined by dividing the nation into MSAs (Metropolitan Statistical Areas). CMS chose 67 MSAs.

Many commenters noted problems for low volume providers, which include primarily the difficulty in investing in the resources to administrate CJR. CMMI will have different target prices for low volume hospitals. Since hip fractures tend to be in low volume settings, these would also have a different target price.

Average and maximum episode payments:

Region	469 Avg	470 Avg	469 High	470 High
New England	$47,928	$24,858	$93,682	$48,433
Middle Atlantic	$52,028	$27,406	$102,359	$55,615
East North Central	$50,954	$25,480	$102,222	$53,548
West North Central	$46,189	$23,800	$100,992	$51,357
South Atlantic	$51,239	$25,989	$106,332	$53,516
East South Central	$50,328	$26,345	$101,762	$55,965
West South Central	$55,448	$27,464	$113,995	$61,418
Mountain	$47,925	$23,734	$99,425	$50,841
Pacific	$48,874	$23,425	$110,168	$50,527

Definition of the Episode of Care

There is a clinical dimension that describes the clinical conditions and associated services that comprise the episode. Hip and knee replacements are the primary focus of the model.

There is a time dimension that describes the beginning, middle, and end of the episode.

Only inpatient joint replacements are covered by CJR.

The following is a summary of procedures of LEJR:

> Total knee replacement
> Partial knee replacement
> Total hip replacement
> Partial hip replacement
> Total ankle replacement
> Resurfacing hip, total, acetabulum and femoral head
> Resurfacing hip, partial, femoral head
> Resurfacing hip, partial, acetabulum
> Lower leg or ankle reattachment
> Thigh reattachment

The acute care hospital stay is called the "anchor hospitalization."

MS-DRG 469 and MS-DRG 470 are the DRG groupings that trigger the episode. MS-466, MS-DRG 467, and MS-DRG 468 are revision codes and are not included in CJR.

Here is further detail from CMS concerning included operating room procedures:

DRG 469 MAJOR JOINT REPLACEMENT OR REATTACHMENT OF LOWER EXTREMITY W MCC
DRG 470 MAJOR JOINT REPLACEMENT OR REATTACHMENT OF LOWER EXTREMITY W/O MCC
OPERATING ROOM PROCEDURES
Replacement of Right Hip Joint with Autologous Tissue Substitute, Open Approach
Replacement of Right Hip Joint with Synthetic Substitute, Metal on Polyethylene, Open Approach
Replacement of Right Hip Joint with Synthetic Substitute, Metal on Metal, Open Approach
Replacement of Right Hip Joint with Synthetic Substitute, Ceramic on Ceramic, Open Approach
Replacement of Right Hip Joint with Synthetic Substitute, Ceramic on Polyethylene, Open Approach
Replacement of Right Hip Joint with Synthetic Substitute, Open Approach
Replacement of Right Hip Joint with Nonautologous Tissue Substitute, Open Approach
Replacement of Right Hip Joint, Acetabular Surface with Autologous Tissue Substitute, Open Approach
Replacement of Right Hip Joint, Acetabular Surface with Synthetic Substitute, Metal, Open Approach
Replacement of Right Hip Joint, Acetabular Surface with Synthetic Substitute, Ceramic, Open Approach
Replacement of Right Hip Joint, Acetabular Surface with Synthetic Substitute, Polyethylene, Open Approach

Replacement of Right Hip Joint, Acetabular Surface with Synthetic Substitute, Open Approach
Replacement of Right Hip Joint, Acetabular Surface with Nonautologous Tissue Substitute, Open Approach
Replacement of Left Hip Joint with Autologous Tissue Substitute, Open Approach
Replacement of Left Hip Joint with Synthetic Substitute, Metal on Polyethylene, Open Approach
Replacement of Left Hip Joint with Synthetic Substitute, Metal on Metal, Open Approach
Replacement of Left Hip Joint with Synthetic Substitute, Ceramic on Ceramic, Open Approach
Replacement of Left Hip Joint with Synthetic Substitute, Ceramic on Polyethylene, Open Approach
Replacement of Left Hip Joint with Synthetic Substitute, Open Approach
Replacement of Left Hip Joint with Nonautologous Tissue Substitute, Open Approach
Replacement of Right Knee Joint with Autologous Tissue Substitute, Open Approach
Replacement of Right Knee Joint with Synthetic Substitute, Open Approach
Replacement of Right Knee Joint with Nonautologous Tissue Substitute, Open Approach
Replacement of Left Knee Joint with Autologous Tissue Substitute, Open Approach
Replacement of Left Knee Joint with Synthetic Substitute, Open Approach
Replacement of Left Knee Joint with Nonautologous Tissue Substitute, Open Approach
Replacement of Left Hip Joint, Acetabular Surface with Autologous Tissue Substitute, Open Approach
Replacement of Left Hip Joint, Acetabular Surface with Synthetic Substitute, Metal, Open Approach
Replacement of Left Hip Joint, Acetabular Surface with Synthetic Substitute, Ceramic, Open Approach
Replacement of Left Hip Joint, Acetabular Surface with Synthetic Substitute, Polyethylene, Open Approach
Replacement of Left Hip Joint, Acetabular Surface with Synthetic Substitute, Open Approach
Replacement of Left Hip Joint, Acetabular Surface with Nonautologous Tissue Substitute, Open Approach
Replacement of Right Ankle Joint with Autologous Tissue Substitute, Open Approach
Replacement of Right Ankle Joint with Synthetic Substitute, Open Approach
Replacement of Right Ankle Joint with Nonautologous Tissue Substitute, Open Approach
Replacement of Left Ankle Joint with Autologous Tissue Substitute, Open Approach
Replacement of Left Ankle Joint with Synthetic Substitute, Open Approach
Replacement of Left Ankle Joint with Nonautologous Tissue Substitute, Open Approach
Replacement of Right Hip Joint, Femoral Surface with Autologous Tissue Substitute, Open Approach
Replacement of Right Hip Joint, Femoral Surface with Synthetic Substitute, Metal, Open Approach
Replacement of Right Hip Joint, Femoral Surface with Synthetic Substitute, Ceramic, Open Approach
Replacement of Right Hip Joint, Femoral Surface with Synthetic Substitute, Open Approach
Replacement of Right Hip Joint, Femoral Surface with Nonautologous Tissue Substitute, Open Approach
Replacement of Left Hip Joint, Femoral Surface with Autologous Tissue Substitute, Open Approach
Replacement of Left Hip Joint, Femoral Surface with Synthetic Substitute, Metal, Open Approach
Replacement of Left Hip Joint, Femoral Surface with Synthetic Substitute, Ceramic, Open Approach
Replacement of Left Hip Joint, Femoral Surface with Synthetic Substitute, Open Approach
Replacement of Left Hip Joint, Femoral Surface with Nonautologous Tissue Substitute, Open Approach
Replacement of Right Knee Joint, Femoral Surface with Autologous Tissue Substitute, Open Approach
Replacement of Right Knee Joint, Femoral Surface with Synthetic Substitute, Open Approach
Replacement of Right Knee Joint, Femoral Surface with Nonautologous Tissue Substitute, Open Approach
Replacement of Left Knee Joint, Femoral Surface with Autologous Tissue Substitute, Open Approach
Replacement of Left Knee Joint, Femoral Surface with Synthetic Substitute, Open Approach
Replacement of Left Knee Joint, Femoral Surface with Nonautologous Tissue Substitute, Open Approach
Replacement of Right Knee Joint, Tibial Surface with Autologous Tissue Substitute, Open Approach
Replacement of Right Knee Joint, Tibial Surface with Synthetic Substitute, Open Approach
Replacement of Right Knee Joint, Tibial Surface with Nonautologous Tissue Substitute, Open Approach
Replacement of Left Knee Joint, Tibial Surface with Autologous Tissue Substitute, Open Approach
Replacement of Left Knee Joint, Tibial Surface with Synthetic Substitute, Open Approach
Replacement of Left Knee Joint, Tibial Surface with Nonautologous Tissue Substitute, Open Approach
Supplement Right Hip Joint with Resurfacing Device, Open Approach
Supplement Right Hip Joint, Acetabular Surface with Resurfacing Device, Open Approach
Supplement Left Hip Joint with Resurfacing Device, Open Approach
Supplement Left Hip Joint, Acetabular Surface with Resurfacing Device, Open Approach
Supplement Right Hip Joint, Femoral Surface with Resurfacing Device, Open Approach
Supplement Left Hip Joint, Femoral Surface with Resurfacing Device, Open Approach
Reattachment of Right Femoral Region, Open Approach

Reattachment of Left Femoral Region, Open Approach
Reattachment of Right Upper Leg, Open Approach
Reattachment of Left Upper Leg, Open Approach
Reattachment of Right Knee Region, Open Approach
Reattachment of Left Knee Region, Open Approach
Reattachment of Right Lower Leg, Open Approach
Reattachment of Left Lower Leg, Open Approach
Reattachment of Right Ankle Region, Open Approach
Reattachment of Left Ankle Region, Open Approach
Reattachment of Right Foot, Open Approach
Reattachment of Left Foot, Open Approach

CMMI decided to risk-stratify the target price for each MS–DRG-anchored episode based on a beneficiary's hip fracture status.

The reason why outpatient LEJR is not covered in CJR is because outpatient LEJR is currently not covered in the outpatient setting. The current CJR ruling reflects current CMS policy. There is an assumption that when CMS IPPS policy changes to allow payment in outpatient settings, then the CJR ruling will be amended. CMMI has recognized that if LEJR moves to the outpatient setting, then the equation for target pricing would probably be affected and new calculations would need to be made.

Related Services Included in the Episode

Items that have historically been part of the episode of MS-DRG 469 and MS-DRG 470 are in the episode. Unrelated items will not be included in the episode. This is important because if an unrelated item occurs in the 90-day, period, it will not be placed in the calculation that goes into the retrospective reconciliation.

Here is a list of the related services:
- Physicians' services.
- Inpatient hospital services (including readmissions), with certain exceptions discussed later in this section.
- Inpatient psychiatric facility (IPF) services.
- Long Term Care Hospital (LTCH) services.
- IRF (Inpatient Rehabilitation Facility) services.
- SNF (Skilled Nursing Facility) services.
- HHA (Home Health Aid) services.
- Hospital outpatient services.
- Independent outpatient therapy services.
- Clinical laboratory services.
- Durable medical equipment (DME).
- Part B drugs.
- Hospice.

CMMI decided to identify the excluded services rather than the included services. This means that essentially all the services in the episode of care period are included unless you have clinical justification to exclude them. The onus, therefore, is on you to anticipate and to clinically justify exclusions.

<u>Understanding Sample Services Included in the Episode</u>

Diagnosis codes directly related to LEJR are included.

Examples of diagnoses that would not be excluded on this basis include surgical site infection and venous thromboembolism.

No claims for services for diagnoses that are related to pre-existing chronic conditions such as diabetes, which may be affected by care furnished during the episode, should be excluded.

Severe exacerbations of most chronic conditions are included especially since some of these readmissions were affected by care during the episode. Effectively, you are responsible for conditions that could have been affected by your care during the episode.

Anticipate that a majority MS–DRGs for readmissions will be included in CJR episodes as related services.

All disease-related surgical MS–DRGs for readmissions, such as hip/knee revision, in CJR episodes.

All body system surgical MS-DRGs such as insertion of a vena cava filter are included.

Pressure ulcers and pre-ulcer skin changes are included.

Chronic diseases are included only if they could have been affected by the episode. CMS generally notes that most chronic diseases are in this category. Chronic anemia appears to be an example of this and is probably included.

All outpatient physical therapy, occupational therapy, and speech services are included.

Inpatient Psychiatric Facility (IPF) admissions are included in the bundle.

Claims for substance abuse and mental health are included.

Hospice services within the 90-day period are included.

DME, even certain prosthetics, braces, and customized DME are included unless they were fashioned for one of the excluded diagnoses.

Part B claims for rheumatoid arthritis treatment, even if pre-dating the episode, are included. The issue of pre-op rheumatoid factors is not an issue because medications are excluded. EM codes of for visits to rheumatologists are included.

Post-acute care (PAC) services are included even if they occur after an excluded readmission.

Part B claims for communication, cognitive, or swallow-related diagnoses are included.

Understanding Sample Services Excluded from the Episode

CJR will exclude only those Medicare Part A and B-covered items and services furnished during the episode that are unrelated to LEJR procedures based on clinical justification, and the exclusions will apply throughout the episode duration.

CJR excluded services for readmission are MS-DRG based and ICD-10 for Part B services.

Hemophilia clotting factors are excluded.

New technology add-on payments for new drugs, technologies, or services are excluded from the calculation of the bundle and will be paid under IPPS. This was so as to not hamper the introduction of these technologies that would benefit patients.

Admissions for oncology and trauma MS–DRGs are excluded.

Surgical MS-DRGs for chronic conditions, such as prostatectomy, are excluded.

Acute disease surgical MS-DRGs, such as appendectomy, are excluded.

Acute disease diagnoses like head trauma are excluded.

Other examples from the exclusion list are: Salmonella, fungal infections, perinatal issues, tuberculosis, infections, STDs, neoplasms, sleep disorders, spinal abscesses, ENT issues, and fractures of the skull, neck, and trunk.

Part D covered drugs are excluded from the episode mainly because enrollment in Part D for patients is voluntary.

Outpatient Prospective Payment System (OPPS) transitional pass-through payments will be excluded. OPPS transitional pass-though items are HCPCS level II codes (C1300-C9899) for biological, devices, and drugs that offer temporary additional payments. Companies submit applications for their products to get this distinction. CMS posts these on their website. Here is a link to a recent PDF list: https://www.cms.gov/Medicare/Medicare-Fee-for-Service-Payment/HospitalOutpatientPPS/Downloads/Complet-list-DeviceCats-OPPS.pdf

Chemotherapy administrative service are excluded.

Chemotherapy and all associated payment codes are excluded based on reporting the correct diagnosis codes.

**

CMMI is not budging in their belief that medical MS-DRGs are linked to the hospitalization for the procedure as a complication of the illness to the surgery, a complication of treatment or interactions with the health care system, or a chronic illness that may have been affected by the course of care. In other words, don't count on getting exclusion through written justifications even though they say that this is theoretically possible.

**

If a patient gets a Hospital Acquired Condition (HAC) during the episode, the hospital acquired condition penalty would not itself inflate the target price such that CMS would pay back the hospital acquired condition penalty through a reconciliation payment.

There are some conditions that CMS, in policies unrelated to this ruling, does not pay for with respect to certain complications and readmissions. CJR does not add new policy to these previous policies.

Duration of Episodes of Care

The episode begins within 3 days prior to and including the date of admission of the anchor hospitalization for MS-DRG 469 and MS-DRG-470. It includes all services based on CMS policies and would include all claims placed by entities wholly owned or wholly operated by the admitting hospital (or another entity under arrangements with the admitting hospital). The episode ends 90 days after discharge. The day of discharge itself counts as the first day of the post-discharge period. Medicare will be monitoring the 30-day post episode time period to check for increased spending to make sure participant hospitals are not delaying appropriate care. This 30-day period is not officially in the episode.

Patients Included:

- Enrolled in Medicare A and B during the entire episode
- Eligibility for Medicare is not based on End Stage Renal Disease (ESRD)
- Beneficiary not enrolled in managed care plans

- Beneficiary not enrolled in United Mine Workers of American health plan
- Medicare must be the primary payer

Even though certain events such as preoperative risk assessment and preoperative testing appear to be related to LEJR, they are not included. The episode initiates on admission with a three-day prior payment window.

There will be risk stratifying of the target price based on the presence or absence of a hip fracture.

While some commenters asked CMS to exclude patients who lived remote from the anchor hospital this was rejected by CMS.

If a physician who opted out of Medicare surgeon does the surgery, the bundle is still executed the same way.

An episode can be cancelled if the beneficiary no longer meets the same inclusion criteria for the beginning of the episode at any point during the episode.

The following circumstances would cancel the episode:

1. The beneficiary is readmitted to an acute care hospital during the episode and discharged again for a second MS-DRG 469 or MS-DRG 470.
2. The beneficiary dies during the anchor hospitalization.
3. The beneficiary initiates an episode under one of the BPCI models.

If a Medicare payment for included services spans a period of care that extends past the end of the episode, then the charges get prorated in the reconciliation.

There are a number of major reasons for readmissions that all CJR participants should know:

- Surgical site infections (18.8 percent).
- Prosthesis issues (7.5 percent).
- Venous thromboembolism (6.3 percent).
- Bleeding (6.3 percent).
- Orthopaedic related (5.1 percent).
- Pulmonary (3.2 percent).
- Cardiac (2.4 percent).
- CNS or CVA (2.4 percent).
- Ileus or Obstruction (2.3 percent).
- Sepsis (2.1 percent).

Participant hospitals will develop the care pathways and partnerships that should be helpful to participant hospitals, such as waivers of Medicare program rules, the opportunity to engage in certain financial arrangements, and the ability to offer certain beneficiary incentives.

Methodology for Setting Episode Prices and Paying Model Participants Under the CJR Model

TABLE 8—PERFORMANCE YEARS FOR CJR MODEL

Year	Calendar year	Episodes included in performance year
1	2016	Episodes that start on or after April 1, 2016, and end on or before December 31, 2016.
2	2017	Episodes that end between January 1, 2017, and December 31, 2017, inclusive.
3	2018	Episodes that end between January 1, 2018, and December 31, 2018, inclusive.
4	2019	Episodes that end between January 1, 2019, and December 31, 2019, inclusive.
5	2020	Episodes that end between January 1, 2020, and December 31, 2020, inclusive.

Retrospective Payment Methodology

All providers and suppliers caring for Medicare beneficiaries in CJR episodes would continue to bill and be paid as usual under the applicable Medicare payment system.

All the claims representing payment performance will be aggregated with episode quality parameters. These will be compared against predefined targets in quality and costs.

After the participant hospital's actual episode performance in quality and spending are compared against the previous episode quality thresholds and target prices, Medicare would make a payment to the hospital (reconciliation payment), unless the hospital owes money to Medicare (resulting in Medicare repayment). Reconciliation payments are not included in setting year-to-year target prices.

The episodes of Year 1 are not included for repayments. Year 2 is phased in. In year 3 hospitals have full responsibility based on a specific schedule.

The payment model does not limit a beneficiary's ability to choose among Medicare providers and suppliers. Beneficiaries can choose providers who have opted out of Medicare with the same costs, copayments, and responsibilities as they have with other Medicare services.

CMS will allow participant hospitals to enter into financial sharing arrangements with certain providers and suppliers (collaborators). Beneficiaries cannot be restricted or directed to these providers. Stark laws need to be followed.

14

TWO SIDED RISK MODEL

Target prices are set for each participant hospital each year.

After adding the Part A and Part B there will be possible adjustments.

1. Certain existing Medicare systems have payment provisions
2. Some service may straddle the episode of care
3. Some high payment episodes may get an adjustment

The hospital performance and reconciliation payments or repayments are independent of, and do not replace special payment provisions. Some of these special payments are:

- HRRP
- HAC
- HIQR
- OQR
- EHR Incentive Program
- DSH
- Uncompensated Care
- IME
- SCHs, MDHs
- IRF QRP
- SNF QRP
- IPF QRP
- HH QRP
- LTCH QRP
- HIV Programs
- ASC QRP
- PQRS
- Physician Value-based Modifier Program

Even though some beneficiaries may exhaust benefits during an episode, beneficiary benefits packages will not be changed by the presence of CJR.

Services that extend beyond the end of the episode will be prorated. The same prorated approach is for services that started before the episode such as home health aides.

For high payment cases, the episode calculation will be capped at 2 times the standard deviation of the target price. This prevents an exceptionally high case from altering an accurate target price in the next year.

Hip fracture cases are calculated differently, with a different target price.

Episode Price Setting Methodology

Each hospital will have eight target prices for years 1,3,4, and 5

MS-DRG	Time Range	Patient-reported Outcomes Submission
469	1/1-9/30	Successful completion
470	1/1/-9/30	Successful completion
469	10/1-12/31	Successful completion
470	10/1-12/31	Successful completion
469	1/1-9/30	Unsuccessful completion
470	1/1/-9/30	Unsuccessful completion
469	10/1-12/31	Unsuccessful completion
470	10/1-12/31	Unsuccessful completion

For year 2, there will be 16 categories to take into account phased payments and repayments.

Three years of historical data are used to calculated target

prices. Some of the pricing calculations will be based on

regional data.

There are no target price adjustments based on risk related to patient-specific factors.

There are no target price adjustments based on Hierarchical Condition Category (HCC) scores.

There are no price adjustments for hip vs. knee replacements.

The ruling to not risk adjust has been recognized as a potential problem and CMS claims to be working on methods to try to risk adjust in the future.

The only price adjustment related to risk is for LEJR for hip fractures.

Summary of Target Price Methodology: Initially, the target price is weighted towards hospital-specific target prices and later, weighted toward regional target process.

Year	Hospital-Specific Weight	Regional Weight	Period
1	2/3	1/3	2012-2014
2	2/3	1/3	2012-2014
3	1/3	2/3	2014-2016
4	0	3/3	2014-2016
5	0	3/3	2016-2018

The use of historical pricing data

CMS will use three years of historical expenditures, updated every other year, to set target prices.

There will be a calculation to mitigate changes in the Medicare payment system by trending the final year of payments and adjusting the first two years.

There are other updates and adjustments that are difficult to calculate yourself as a hospital but are designed to take into account Medicare updated payments so the target price can have the proper validity.

Medicare will also have complex equations to update for factors related to the acute care hospital, physician services, SNF, HHA, and other services.

There will also be adjustments to the hospital-specific price based on regional data. CMS anticipates that regional pricing will be the only way to set target prices in the future- by year 4. This will be especially true with low volume hospitals, which will have their prices determined by regional data.

Target prices are also adjusted relative to the participant hospital's wage index.

Medicare is taking a further 2% discount off the top of the target price to take advantage of anticipated savings.

Quality Parameters

Participant hospitals are incentivized to improve quality through collecting quality performance measures. CJR uses two quality measures- standardized complication rate after hip and knee arthroplasty (NQF #1550) and Hospital Consumer Assessment of Healthcare Providers and Systems Survey measure (NQF #0166). Quality performance points are variable that modify the repayment and the reconciliation payment. While the NQF #1550 is a measure of the performance of the joint replacement service, the NQF #0166 (HCAHPS) is a hospital-wide measure. This is important to keep in mind as non-orthopaedic services, because of this, impact significantly on CJR through this measure.

If the actual spending is less than the target price, then quality parameters must be met to receive reconciliation payments.

Hospitals must meet or exceed the measure reporting thresholds RSCR & HCAHPS) to be eligible for a reconciliation payment.

CMS will use a 3-year rolling performance or applicable period for these required measures.

To link to the following parameters go to www.qualityforum.org and search for these forms.

Hospital-level RSCR following elective primary THA and/or TKA (NQF #1550):

HCAHPS Survey measure (NQF#0166):

Approach to Combine Pricing Features

1. Calculate historical CJR episode payments for the last 3-historical years.
2. Remove effects of special payment provisions.
3. Prorate Medicare payments for episode services that precede the beginning or extend past the end of the episode.
4. Normalize for wage adjustment variation.
5. Trend forward 2 oldest historical years to the most recent year. Take into account hip fracture status.
6. Cap high episode payment episodes with payment ceilings.
7. Calculate participant hospital and region-specific weights to determine historical average payments.
8. Calculate weighted factors.
9. Blend together each hospital-specific updated, pooled, historical average episode with region-specific payments. Hospitals with low volume will use region-specific data.
10. Reintroduce hospital-specific wage variations and normalization factors.
11. Multiply the appropriate discount factor.
12. Multiply the MS-DRG anchored episode prices by an anchor factor to determine MS-DRG 469 target prices.

Voluntary Patient-Reported Outcome (PRO) Measure

CMS has a measure in development called "The Hospital-Level Performance Measure(s) of Patient-Reported Outcomes Following Elective THA or TKA." The shorthand for this is the "THA/TKA patient-reported outcome measure."

At the current time, 2016, hospitals will not be financially accountable for the patient-reported outcomes measures. There would be a benefit to reporting these voluntary measures because if you do, there will be a reduction in the 2.0% discount to 1.7%. This 0.3% reduction is called the "voluntary reporting payment adjustment." CMS calculates that the .3% reduction is worth $75.00/episode, which will pay for collecting the outcomes on a single episode. Effectively, there is only an upside to this provision.

CMS assigns the participant hospital measure value to a performance percentile and then quality performance points are assigned based on the following performance percentile scale:

> 10.00 points for 90th.
> 9.25 points for 80th and <90th.
> 8.50 points for 70th and <80th;
> 7.75 points for 60th and <70th.
> 7.00 points for 50th and <60th.
> 6.25 points for 40th and <50th.
> 5.50 points for 30th and <40th.
> 0.0 points for <30th.

For the Hospital Consumer Assessment of Healthcare Providers and Systems Survey measure (NQF #0166) described in § 510.400(a)(2), CMS assigns the participant hospital measure value to a performance percentile and quality performance points are assigned based on the following performance percentile scale:

> 8.00 points for 90th.
> 7.40 points for 80th and <90th.
> 6.80 points for 70th and <80th.
> 6.20 points for 60th and <70th.
> 5.60 points for 50th and <60th.
> 5.00 points for 40th and <50th.
> 4.40 points for 30th and <40th.
> 0.0 points for <30th.

Methodology to Determine Performance on Quality Measures

Performance on the required measures for each hospital will be compared to national data obtained through HIQR (Hospital Inpatient Quality Reporting). Most acute care hospitals already participate in this system.

For the voluntary patient-reported outcomes measures, hospitals must meet all of the following:

1. Submit all the required data elements
2. 80% collection rate of all eligible THA/TKA patients
3. Submission must occur within 60 days of the end of the performance period

Methodology to Link Quality and Payment

Minimal thresholds of quality are required.

Success in quality has two advantages:

1. You are eligible for reconciliation payments. If you don't meet quality standards, even if you save money, you will not get reconciliation payments.
2. You are eligible for a reduction in the 2.0% discount to 1.7%

> It is important to note that while you can spend a lot of effort figuring out all the various scoring, it would be best to focus your resources on preventing readmissions, lowering complications, and increasing patient satisfaction.

CMS will be using results generated from the HIQR program posted on Hospital Compare, *https:// data.medicare.gov/data/hospital-compare*) for the HIQR Program.

After many comments CMS has determined:

QUALITY MEASURE WEIGHTS UNDER THE COMPOSITE QUALITY SCORE

Quality Measure	Weight in Composite Quality Score (%)
NQF #1550	50
NQF #0166	40
Voluntary PRO (Patient-Reported Outcomes	10

Quality Composite Score and Payment

Score Range	Category	Eligible	Discount for Reconciliation Payment	Discount for Repayment
>13.2	Excellent	Yes	1.5%	Y1: N/A Y2-3: 0.5% Y4-5: 1.5%
≥6 and <13.2	Good	Yes	3%	Y1: N/A Y2-3: 1% Y4-5: 2%
≥6 and <6	Acceptable	Yes	3%	Y1: N/A Y2-3: 2% Y4-5: 3%
<4	Below Acceptable	No	3%	Y1: N/A Y2-3: 2% Y4-5: 3%

At this time, 2016, the readmission quality parameter (NQF #1551) is removed from the final composite quality score.

There are quality improvement points for hospitals that show substantial improvement in quality. "Substantial" is defined as improving 3 deciles.

Summary:

1. CMS will use a composite quality score.
2. The score is based on NQF #1550 (complications), NQF #0116 (HCAHPS), and the submission of THA/TKA voluntary PRO.
3. These will be summarized in four categories
4. Below Acceptable
5. Acceptable
6. Good
7. Excellent
8. "Composite Quality Score" means a score computed for each hospital to summarize its level of performance(composite quality scores links quality to payment)
9. Hospitals are assigned a composite quality score each year based on their performance and improvement on the two quality measures:
   A.THA/TKA complication measure (NQF 1550).
   B. HCAHPS measure (NQF 0166)
Performance and improvement in the PRO data are not taken into consideration as finalized in the rule. However, successful submission of the PRO data will contribute to increase the composite quality score.
10. "Quality Improvement Points" are points added if the hospital's performance percentage on an individual quality measure increases from the previous year by at least 3 deciles.

Process for Reconciliation

CMS will calculate the Net Payment Reconciliation Amount (NPRA).

Reconciliation payments are not included as Medicare payments. This would be adding the reconciliation payments to the anchor hospitalization costs.

In summary, after the completion of a performance year, each hospital's actual payment performance will be compared to target prices creating the raw NPRA. This will be adjusted for the stop-loss and stop-gain limits, as well as post-episode spending. This creates the NPRA.

CMS anticipates this reconciliation to take place 2 months after the end of the performance year. Reconciliation payments or repayments will be distributed in

Quarter 2 in the year after the performance year. Other CMS incentive programs will be reconciled a second time- 14 months after the end of the performance year. RAC (Recovery Audit Contractor) and MAC reviews are still in place irrespective of timing of CJR.

TABLE 22—SAMPLE RECONCILIATION RESULTS

	Performance Year 1 (2016) raw NPRA	Performance Year 1 subsequent reconciliation calculation	Difference between PY1 subsequent reconciliation calculation and raw NPRA	Performance Year 2 (2017) raw NPRA	Reconciliation payment made to hospital in quarter 2 2018
Hospital A	$50,000	$40,000	($10,000)	$25,000	$15,000

TABLE 24—FINAL TIMEFRAME FOR RECONCILIATION IN CJR

Model performance year	Model performance period	Reconciliation claims submitted by	Reconciliation payment or repayment	Second calculation to address overlaps and claims run-out	Second calculation adjustment to reconciliation amount
Year 1 *	Episodes ending June 30, 2016 to December 31, 2016.	March 1, 2017 ....|	Q2 2017	March 1, 2018	Q2 2018.
Year 2	Episodes ending January 1, 2017 through December 31, 2017.	March 1, 2018	Q2 2018	March 1, 2019	Q2 2019.
Year 3	Episodes ending January 1, 2018 through December 31, 2018.	March 1, 2019	Q2 2019	March 2, 2020	Q2 2020.
Year 4	Episodes ending January 1, 2019 through December 31, 2019.	March 2, 2020	Q2 2020	March 1, 2021	Q2 2021.
Year 5	Episodes ending January 1, 2020 through December 31, 2020.	March 1, 2021	Q2 2021	March 1, 2022	Q2 2022.

* Note that the reconciliation for Year 1 would not include repayment responsibility from CJR hospitals.

Overlaps with other CMS Savings Programs

There are a number of programs that overlap.

Program	Description	Shared Savings?	Per-beneficiary-per-month payments
Pioneer ACO	ACO	Yes	No
Medicare Shared Savings Program	ACO	Yes	No
Next Generation ACO Model	ACO	Yes	No
CPCi	Pay for improvement	Yes	Yes
MAPCP	Medical Homes	Yes	Yes
BPCI	Bundled Payment	No	No
OCM	Oncology	No	Yes
CEC	ACO for ESRD	Yes	No
Million Hearts	Heart/Stroke	No	Yes
MCCM	Hospice	No	Yes

Specifically for BPCI, the BPCI takes precedence over CJR or any portion of CJR.

If an ACO is involved, the reconciliation payment goes to the participating hospital and not the ACO.

ACO's cannot opt out of CJR.

ACO's cannot steer patients to their own providers.

There are a few Per Beneficiary Per Month(PBPM) programs. CMS will determine payments on a model-to-model basis. If you are in one of these programs, contact CMS directly. PBPM payments during the bundle are included in all calculations.

Limits on Adjustment Financial Responsibilities

The amount of repayment is limited.

The stop-loss limit on repayment is 5% of the NPRA (effectively the target price) in year 2 and 10% in year 3, and 20% in years 4 and 5.

An example of this is as follows:

In year 3, a hospital has 10 episodes with a target price of $50,000/episode. The actual claims data show $650,000. This is a total of $150,000 over spend. Since the total target should have been $500,000 then 10% of this is $50,000, which is the maximum amount of repayment.

Limit on Reconciliation Payments

To prevent improper incentives to cut services to save money, CMS has put stop- gains on the repayments.

Year 1,2- 5%
Year 3- 10%
Year 4,5- 20%

Stop-loss limits are the same except in year 1 when there is no repayment.

Policies for Certain Hospitals to Limit Repayment Responsibility

Certain hospitals have lower risk tolerance and less infrastructure to support CJR. This mainly applies to rural hospitals.

Spending Percentages of Inpatient and SNF

	MS-DRG 469	MS-DRG-470
Inpatient	53%	55%
SNF	27%	18%

Sole Community Hospitals (SCH) and Medicare Dependent Hospitals (MDH), and

Rural Referral Centers (RRC) will have repayment protections. These have specific definitions that are obtained at the CMS website. Hospitals need to apply for these statuses through their MAC (Medicare Administrative Contractor). CMS is finalizing a lower stop-loss for these hospitals.

Hospital Responsibility for Increased Post-Episode Expenses

There is concern that a hospital will withhold or delay medically necessary care until after the episode ends. To mitigate this, CMS will calculate the 30-day post-discharge claims of CJR-included and CJR-excluded events. If a hospital incurs more than 3 standard deviations from the regional average, then the hospital will need to repay that amount with the standard stop-loss provisions.

Appeals

Hospitals can appeal reconciliation payments and repayments.

If hospitals do not repay the amount they owe, then past and future Medicare payments will be used to recoup this money.

Only hospitals can initiate an appeal or a dispute resolution process.

Hospitals have 45 days to submit a calculation error appeal.

Financial Arrangements and Beneficiary Incentives

Hospitals can engage with Collaborators to share the reconciliation payments , the internal cost savings, and bear some of the repayments costs. These collaborators can also invest in infrastructure to develop programs to deploy CJR. Hospitals define these arrangements.

These CJR Collaborators include:

- SNFs
- HHAs
- LTCHs
- IRFs
- PGPs
- Physicians, non-physician practitioners, and providers of physical therapy services

CMS believes these collaborators should have responsibility for investing in processes to improve the episode of care.

All collaborators must furnish services directly to Medicare beneficiaries to be eligible.

The arrangement is called a "CJR Sharing Arrangement." The arrangements must be in writing and are referred to as "Participation Agreements."

Three things can be shared:

1. Reconciliation payments
2. Internal cost savings
3. Responsibility for repayment

The payment to a collaborator is called a "gain-sharing payment."

Gain sharing arrangements must be related to contributions to care redesign and must directly be for treated CJR patients. This involvement status is auditable by HHS. Medicare will not be screening CJR collaborators.

CJR collaborators and agreements must contain the following as a minimum:

1. A specific methodology to calculate and verify internal cost savings through these gain-sharing arrangements (due to redesign). These are cost savings attributable only to the hospital. This does not include cost savings realized by the collaborator.
2. A description of the methodology for determining the percentage or dollar amount that will be paid to the collaborator.
3. A description of how these payments will be made.
4. A description of how the hospital and collaborator will share repayments to Medicare.
5. Collaborators must not have opted out of Medicare.
6. Sharing arrangements must be in place before care is initiated.
7. The hospital must keep records concerning the criteria in selection of collaborators and their contribution to quality care. The selection criteria cannot be based directly or indirectly on the volume or value of referrals.
8. The quality criteria in judging the collaborator must be related to the episode of care.
9. If the collaborator in a calendar year does not meet these quality criteria, then they are not eligible for gain sharing payments.
10. Hospitals must keep accurate documentation of the agreements.
11. Hospitals must keep an accurate list of collaborators.
12. The list of collaborators must be open to the public on the hospital's web site.
13. Payments must be made in compliance of fraud and abuse laws. Payments to collaborators for substandard care in CJR episodes or other integrity problems must not be made.
14. Gain sharing payments cannot be made if sharing agreements are not in place.
15. CMS can review all sharing arrangements.

16. Notwithstanding any sharing agreement, the hospital bears all responsibility for full compliance with CJR.
17. The hospital must update its compliance program to include oversight of these arrangements.
18. The board of the hospital or other governing body has overseeing responsibility.
19. Hospitals must have written policies that govern all aspects of the relationship with collaborators. These policies must include provision for collaborators to have met or agree to have met quality criteria for inclusion in gain sharing.
20. An individual's participation as a collaborator must be voluntary, without penalty for non-participation.
21. Gain sharing payments must:
    a. Be solely derived from reconciliation payments and/or internal cost savings.
    b. Be actually and proportionally related to the care of beneficiaries in the CJR.
    c. Be distributed annually.
    d. Not be loans, advance payments, or payments for referrals or other business.
22. Alignment payments (payments that the collaborator pays to the hospital for CJR repayments):
    a. May be made at any interval decided by the parties.
    b. May not be issued prior to a reconciliation report from CMS
    c. May not be a loan, advance payments, or payments for referrals or other business.
23. Payments to collaborators cannot be for non-compliance with fraud and abuse laws or for substandard care.
24. The aggregate amount a hospital can pay a collaborator cannot be more than the hospital received in reconciliation payments.
25. The aggregate amount of all collaborator alignment payments cannot exceed more than 50% of the hospital's repayment.
26. The aggregate amount of alignment payments from any one collaborator must not exceed more than 25% of the hospital repayment.
27. A sharing arrangement must not induce any party to reduce or limit medically necessary services.
28. A sharing agreement cannot restrict a collaborator to make decisions in the best interest of the patient including selection of devices, supplies, and treatments.
29. The methodology of gain sharing must be, in part, based on quality and cannot be related to the volume or value of referrals.
30. Alignment payments cannot be related to the volume or value of referrals.
31. The total amount of gain sharing to a physician in a calendar year cannot be more that 50% of the total Medicare approved amounts under the Physician Fee Schedule.
32. The total amount of gain sharing to a PGP (Physician Group Practice) in a calendar year cannot be more that 50% of the total Medicare approved

amounts under the Physician Fee Schedule.

33. The hospital's determination of internal cost savings must satisfy the following criteria:
    a. Calculated using accepted accounting principles and Government Auditing Standards.
    b. Must be actual cost savings realized by redesign and not realized by any individual or party that is not the hospital.
    c. Cannot be from "paper" savings from accounting conventions or past investment in fixed costs.

34. Payments from collaborators to hospitals can only be in the form of alignment payments.

35. All gain sharing and alignment payments must be made via electronic transfers.

36. All agreements with collaborators must have:
    a. Language that confirms all the features of the gain sharing and alignment payments noted above.
    b. Actual care redesign plans.
    c. A description of how success will be measured.
    d. Management and staffing that will be primarily carrying out changes to care under the CJR model.
    e. A requirement that the collaborator follows all the provisions of CJR.
    f. Provisions that the collaborator agrees to have a compliance program.
    g. Methodology for calculating internal cost savings.
    h. A provision to recoup money from the collaborator in cases of overpayment or fraud.

37. The collaborator that signed the agreement can only make alignment payments.

38. Sharing agreements cannot include any parts that are not alignment payments or gain sharing payments.

39. Agreements must obligate the collaborator to allow access by the hospital and HHS to audit all aspects of the records. This includes site visits.

40. Records must be maintained for 10 years.

41. PGPs have no requirement to distribute gain sharing payments to specific physicians

42. If PGPs choose to give distributions to physicians and non-physician providers, these must be people who participated directly with the care of patients in the CJR.

43. In PGPs, the distribution to an individual cannot exceed 50% of the Physician Fee Schedule and follow the other provisions listed above.

Beneficiary Incentives

Hospitals can furnish certain items and services to engage patients to improve care.
- The incentive must be provided to the beneficiary during the episode of care.
- There must be a reasonable connection between the item or service and the beneficiary's medical care.

- It must be a preventive care or item or service that advances a clinical goal for the beneficiary.
- The cost of the incentive cannot be shifted to another federal program.
- An example is post-surgical monitoring equipment but not technology unrelated to care.
- Items and services must not exceed $1000.00.
- Items of technology over $100.00 are owned by the hospital and must be returned at the end of the episode.
- These items must be the minimum necessary.
- These items and services may be provided by agents under the control of the hospital.
- Items and services cannot be tied to receipt from a particular provider or supplier.
- These items and services cannot be advertised.
- Items or services over $25.00 must be documented.

Waiver of Medicare Program Rules

Certain Medicare program rules will need to be waived to give hospitals flexibility to save money and increase quality.

Waiver:

Home Visits: For CJR post- discharge home visits CMS will waive the "incident to " direct physician supervision rule for physician services.

Allow clinical staff of a physician or non physician practitioner to furnish a visit in the beneficiary's home under the general supervision of a physician.

Permitted only for beneficiaries who do not qualify for Medicare coverage of home health services, patient who are not home bound(Home bound beneficiaries are qualified for Medicare coverage of home health services.)

Allow a maximum of 9 visits during the episode

Billing and payments for Telehealth Services: CMS is waving the geographic site requirements that limit Telehealth payment to services in specific geographic areas or an area in the telemedicine demonstration project. CMS is developing 9 new HCPCS codes for billing of these Telehealth visits in during the episode. These are G9481 through G9489.

Telehealth cannot substitute for home health visits. Telehealth by social workers are not permitted because social work is part of home health services. Telehealth for home health certification needs to be separate and distinct from home health services. Home health services must be face-to-face.

The Telehealth waiver applies to services by physicians and practitioners currently eligible to furnish Medicare-approved telehealth services under the MPFS.

Important Note: If a level 4 or 5 home telehealth visit is claimed and a post-op visit is not claimed, then justification will be required before payment of a level 4 or 5 visit is done.

No additional payments are being made through this waiver to cover setup, equipment costs, or training.

SNF 3-Day Rule

The problem: If Medicare beneficiaries are discharged prior to 3 days of a hospital stay, then Medicare rules stipulate that the Medicare coverage for the SNF is eliminated.

Medicare will waive the SNF 3-day rule years 2-5. The waiver is for 3 star SNFs of the 5-Star Rating System for SNFs on the Nursing Home Compare web site for at least 7 of the last 12 months or better. The receiving SNF would insert a "Treatment Authorization Code" on the claim to receive a waiver.

Enforcement

CMS will apply enforcement mechanisms only to participant hospitals. It will use these mechanisms:

- Does not comply with the CJR.
- Non-compliant with CMS, HHS, and OIG monitoring
- Participant hospitals are responsible not only for their own compliance but those of their collaborating entities. CMS can take remedial action against a participating hospital for actions of a collaborating entity.
- This may include requiring the participant hospital to terminate the collaborator agreement.

Examples of enforcing mechanisms:

- Warning letter
- Corrective Action Plan
- Reduction or elimination of reconciliation amount
- Termination from the model:
    - Can be for threatening the health and safety of patients.
    - Is subject to sanctions of final action from an accrediting organization.
    - Can be for taking any action CMS feels is not in the best interests of the integrity of CJR.
    - Can be for being subject to action by HHS, OIG, or CMS.
    - Can be for being subject to self-referral violations.

- Can be for CMS not having funds for CJR.
- Can be if CJR is not subject to administrative or judicial review

Quality Measures

Resource: Medicare Hospital Quality Chartbook (https://www.cms.gov/Medicare/ Quality-Initiatives-Patient-Assessment- Instruments/HospitalQualityInits/ OutcomeMeasures.html). This annual Chartbook provides new information about recent trends and variation in condition specific and surgical procedure outcomes by location, hospital characteristics, and patient disparities.

To answer the concern that surgeons may choose to not operate on patients with higher comorbidities, the THA/TKA Readmissions measure (NQF #1551) does a risk adjustment.

For patient-related and reported factors, the HCAHPS Survey measure (NQF #0166) and the Hip disability and Osteoarthritis Outcome Score (HOOS) and the Knee injury and Osteoarthritis Outcome Score (KOOS) address the perspective of the patient.

The current set of outcomes is hospital-centric which encourage collaboration and continues to be in line with the CJR model that the hospital is financially responsible. CMS recognizes there are gaps in choosing the measure relative to the care given in other settings. CMS plans to make more measures that assess the post-acute care setting (PAC).

If hospitals want their own assessments of collaborators, CMS has used the following other measures currently not included in CJR:

- IRF Program Web site at: *https:// www.cms.gov/Medicare/Quality- Initiatives-Patient- Assessment- Instruments/IRF-Quality-Reporting/ index.html*
- Long-Term Care Hospital Quality Reporting Program Web site at: *https://www.cms.gov/Medicare/Quality- Initiatives- Patient-Assessment- Instruments/LTCH- Quality-Reporting/ index.html?redirect=/LTCH-Quality- Reporting/*
- Skilled Nursing Facility Quality initiative Web site at: *https://www.cms.gov/Medicare/Quality- Initiatives-Patient- Assessment- Instruments/NursingHomeQualityInits/ SNF- Quality- Reporting.html*
- Home Health Agencies please see: *https://www. medicare.gov/homehealthcompare/)*
- Nursing Homes please see "about the data" tab at *https://www. medicare.gov/nursinghomecompare/*

CJR performance will be posted on the Hospital Compare web site, http://www.hospitalcompare.hhs.gov.

Quality Measures for Performance Year 1 and Subsequent Years

Historically, the RSCR (Risk-Standardized Complication Rate), NQF #1550, was an average of 4.2 percent with a range of 2.2 to 8.9. In 2011, those numbers increased with an average of 3.1% and a range from 1.4 percent to 6.9%.

For the quality outcomes measure NQF #1550 inclusion, the index admission is the hospitalization that the complication is attributable to.

In summary, as per the use of the complication measure, index admissions are for the following:

- Enrolled in Medicare FFS
- Aged 65 or older
- Enrolled in Part A and Part B for the 12 months prior to the date of the index admission and during
- Having a primary THA/TKA without any of the following:
    o Femur, hip, or pelvic fracture coded as primary or secondary field
    o Partial hip arthroplasty (PHA)
    o Revision procedures with concurrent THA/TKA
    o Mechanical complications coded in the primary diagnosis
    o Malignant neoplasm
    o Removal of implanted devices
    o Transfer to another acute care facility for THA/TKA
- Exclude:
    o Patients who signed out AMA
    o Admissions for patients with more than two THA/TKA codes during the index hospitalization
    o Patient without at least 90 days post-discharge Medicare FFS enrollment

There will be a risk adjustment based on hospital case mix.

In calculating the Risk Standardized Complication Rate (RSCR), the predicted vs. the actual will be compared.

There will be no socioeconomic risk adjustment done at this time.

Risk-Standardized Readmission Rate (NQF #1551) will be used to assess this issue.

It is important to keep in mind that Part A and Part B claims are the source of the data for CJR.

Readmissions within 30 days are not eligible to be index admissions. That means that a staged bilateral THA/TKA done within 30 days is considered a readmission and not a second index CJR admission.

Keep in mind: While hip fractures are part of CJR in general the readmissions measures for these diagnoses are not included in RSRR measures.

IMPORTANT NOTE: CMS recognizes there are issues surrounded by the NQF #1551, the readmissions measure and is not finalizing it for the complications sections of CJR model at this time.

The Role of HCAHPS

CMS will be incorporating HCAHPS into quality measures in CJR.

HCAHPS are not being adjusted for socioeconomic status.

Even though the following is recognized, it is not changing the use of HCAHPS
- Hospitals with admission from the ED have different HCAHPS
- Surgical patients are not particularly selected in HCAHPS

Possible New Outcomes Measures

CMS wants Patient-Reported Outcomes Measures (PROM) to be less burdensome and does not want them to be based on proprietary instruments. CMS rejected established joint registries.

The following table summarizes:

1. Demographic, Medicare, and identifier information
2. PROMIS Global for THA/TKA
3. VR-12
4. HOOS
5. KOOS
6. Home support
7. Chronic narcotics
8. ASA
9. Charnley Classification
10. Some history and physical exam findings

Proposed voluntary PRO * and risk variable data elements	Finalized PRO and risk variable data elements	Definition of finalized PRO and risk variable data elements	Timing of collection
Age	N/A	(Will be captured by linking to claims data).	N/A.
Date of Birth **	Date of Birth	(MM/DD/YYYY)	¥90 to 0 days prior to and 270 to 365 days after THA/TKA proce- dure (to be used for linking to claims data).
Gender	N/A	(Will be captured by linking to claims data).	N/A.
Race and Ethnicity **	Race and Ethnicity	Race: American Indian or Alaska Native, Asian, Black or African American, Native Hawaiian or Other Pacific Islander, White.	¥90 to 0 days prior to THA/TKA procedure.
		Ethnicity: Hispanic or Latino, Not Hispanic or Latino.	N/A.
THA or TKA procedure	N/A	(Will be captured as possible by linking to claims data).	270 to 365 days after THA/TKA procedure (to be used for link- ing to claims data).
Date of admission to anchor hos- pitalization**.	Date of admission to anchor hos- pitalization.	(MM/DD/YYYY)	N/A.
Date of discharge from anchor hospitalization.	N/A	(Will be captured as possible by linking to claims data).	270 to 365 days after THA/TKA procedure (to be used for link- ing to claims data).
Date of eligible THA/TKA proce- dure**.	Date of eligible THA/TKA proce- dure.	(MM/DD/YYYY)	¥90 to 0 days prior to and 270 to 365 days after THA/TKA proce- dure (to be used for linking to claims data).
Medicare Health Insurance Claim Number**.	Unique Identifier	Medicare Health Insurance Claim Number.	¥90 to 0 days prior to and 270 to 365 days after THA/TKA proce- dure.
		VR–12 OR PROMIS-Global	¥90 to 0 days prior to and 270 to 365 days after THA/TKA proce- dure.
PROMIS Global (all items)	Generic PROM Instrument for THA and TKA Procedures.	VR–12 OR PROMIS-Global	¥90 to 0 days prior to and 270 to 365 days after TKA procedure.
VR–12 (all items.)	Generic PROM Instrument for THA and TKA Procedures.	KOOS Jr. Only OR KOOS Stiff- ness Subscale AND KOOS Pain Subscale AND KOOS Function, Daily Living Subscale.	¥90 to 0 days prior to and 270 to 365 days after THA procedure.
For TKA patients Knee injury and Osteoarthritis Outcome Score (KOOS[75]) (all items).	Knee-Specific PROM Instrument for TKA Procedures.	HOOS Jr. Only OR HOOS Pain Subscale AND HOOS Function, Daily Living Subscale.	¥90 to 0 days prior to THA/TKA procedure.
For THA patients Hip disability and Osteoarthritis Outcome Score (HOOS[76]) (all items).	Hip-Specific PROM Instrument for THA Procedures.	Body Mass Index (or height in cm and weight in kg).	N/A.
Body Mass Index **	Body Mass Index (or height in cm and weight in kg).	(Will be captured by linking to claims data).	¥90 to 0 days prior to THA/TKA procedure.
Presence of live-in home support, including spouse.	N/A	Provider-reported yes/no ... N/A	N/A.
Use of chronic (≥90 day) nar- cotics**.	Pre-operative use of narcotics	(Will be captured by linking to claims data).	N / A .
American Society of Anesthesiol- ogists (ASA) physical status classification.	N/A	"What amount of pain have you experienced in the last week in your other knee/hip?" (none, mild, moderate, severe, ex- treme).[95]	N / A .
Charnley Classification	N/A	"My BACK PAIN at the moment is" (none, very mild, moderate, fairly severe, very severe, worst imaginable).[96][97]	¥90 to 0 days prior to THA/TKA procedure.
Presence of retained hardware	N/A	N/A	¥90 to 0 days prior to THA/TKA procedure.
Total painful joint count [94]**	Patient-Reported Pain in Non-op- erative Lower Extremity Joint.	N/A	N/A.
		N/A	N / A .
Quantified spinal pain **	Patient-Reported Back (Oswestry Index question).		N / A .

CMS is looking for changes in preoperative and postoperative patient-reported outcomes separately or as a composite measure in THA/TKA.

The preoperative collection phase will be 0-90 days preoperatively and the postoperative data collection phase will be 270-365 days after surgery.

Risk adjustment in the PRO measure has yet to be determined.

Reporting periods are different based on the year.

Successful completion of the voluntary data (PRO)

This depends on:
- Submission of all the data elements
- Must include at least 80% of eligible patients
- Must be within 60 days of the most recent data collection period
- For Year 1, only preoperative data and 50% of eligible patients or 50 eligible patients
- For Years 2-5, need preoperative, postoperative, and 80% of eligible patients
- Submission within 60 days of the most recent reporting period

Finalized Performance Periods and Requirements

The following chart summarizes the percentage completion per year as well as what is required.

Model year	Performance period	Duration of the perform-	Patient population eligible for THA/TKA	Requirements for successful THA/TKA voluntary data submission
2016	July 1, 2016 through August 31, 2016.	2 months	All patients undergoing elective primary THA/TKA procedures performed between July 1, 2016 and August 31, 2016.	Submit PRE-operative data on primary elective THA/TKA procedures for ≥50% or ≥50 eligible procedures performed be- tween July 1, 2016 and August 31, 2016.
2017	July 1, 2016 through August 31, 2016.	13 months ...		Submit POST-operative data on primary elective THA/TKA procedures for ≥50% or ≥50 eligible procedures performed be- tween July 1, 2016 through August 31, 2016.
2017	September 1, 2016 through June 30, 2017.	....	All patients undergoing elective primary THA/TKA procedures performed between July 1, 2016 through August 31, 2016.	Submit PRE-operative data on primary elective THA/TKA procedures for ≥60% or ≥75 procedures performed between September 1, 2016 through June 30, 2017.
2018		22 months ...		Submit POST-operative data on primary elective THA/TKA procedures for ≥60% or ≥75 procedures performed between September 1, 2016 and June 30, 2017.
2018	September 1, 2016 through June 30, 2017.		All patients undergoing elective primary THA/TKA procedures performed between September 1, 2016 through June 30, 2017.	Submit PRE-operative data on primary elective THA/TKA procedures for ≥70% or ≥100 procedures performed between July 1, 2017 and June 30, 2018.
2019	July 1, 2017 through June 30, 2018.	24 months ...		Submit POST-operative data on primary elective THA/TKA procedures for ≥70% or ≥100 procedures performed between July 1, 2017 and June 30, 2018.
2019		....	All patients undergoing elective primary THA/TKA procedures performed between September 1, 2016 and June 30, 2017.	Submit PRE-operative data on primary elective THA/TKA procedures for ≥80% or ≥200 procedures performed between July 1, 2018 and June 30, 2019.
2020	July 1, 2017 through June 30, 2018.	24 months ...		
2020	July 1, 2018 through June 30, 2019.		All patients undergoing elective primary THA/TKA procedures performed between	Submit POST-operative data on primary elective THA/TKA procedures for ≥80% or ≥200 procedures performed between July 1, 2018 and June 30, 2019.

Shared Decision-Making Measure

There has been no decision make by CMS in regard to a measure for shared decision-making, but it is high on their list because they want to use it to manage appropriate care and prevent unnecessary joint replacements from being done. Currently (2016) they are considering such a measure and will do this using the notice-and-comment rulemaking method.

Care Planning Measure

This has not been determined and they will do this using the notice-and-comment rulemaking method.

Use of IT and Health Information Exchange Measures

As the Office of Health Information Technology (OHIT) has already addressed much of this, despite recognition that this is important, there are no measures proposed in CJR for information technology.

The Form, Manner, and Timing of Data Submission of Measures

The two major measures that were adopted by CJR are to be submitted through the existing HIQR (Health Information Quality Reporting) program. These two are:

1. THA/TKA Complications Measure (NQF #1550)
2. HCAHPS Survey Measure (NQF #0166)

The Readmissions measure NQF # 1551 is not being adopted by CJR.

For the PRO (Patient-Reported Outcome) measures, which at this time are voluntary, CJR is not certifying vendors and has taken the position that hospitals can collect the data in any manner they choose. CJR is planning to develop online tools to support this.

SUMMARY OF FINALIZED QUALITY MEASURE PERFORMANCE PERIODS BY YEAR OF THE CJR MODEL

Measure title	CJR Model year				
	1st	2nd	3rd	4th	5th
THA/TKA Complications	April 1, 2013–March 31, 2016.	April 1, 2014–March 31, 2017.	April 1, 2015–March 31, 2018.	April 1, 2016–March 31, 2019.	April 1, 2017–March 31, 2020.
HCAHPS **	July 1, 2015–June 30, 2016.	July 1, 2016–June 30, 2017.	July 1, 2017–June 30, 2018.	July 1, 2018–June 30, 2019.	July 1, 2019–June 30, 2020.

Reporting of Measure Publically

Reporting of two chosen measure results will be on Hospital Compare website. http://www.hosptialcompare.hhs.gov. Hospitals that voluntarily report functional status of the patient will show an icon on the website indicating that. CMS will not report the actual data. Currently CMS is developing this measure. It is called: Hospital-Level Performance Measure(s) of Patient-Reported Outcomes Following Elective Primary Total Hip and/or Total Knee Arthroplasty.

Data Sharing

CMS plans to share selected claims data on beneficiaries in accordance with established security and privacy protections. They recognize that hospital will have their own methods of evaluating performance of CJR as well.

CMS will make this data available in two formats as some hospitals have the ability to analyze raw claims data and some do not.

For those who cannot analyze raw claims data, CMS will provide summary beneficiary claims data reports on the use of healthcare services during all the appropriate periods of care.

These summary reports will provide tools to monitor, understand, and manage utilization and expenditure patterns so they can respond and develop appropriate programs and services.

For hospitals with the capacity to analyze raw claims data, this will be sent in a flat binary format.

Information subject to regulations of alcohol and drug abuse records will be excluded.

Aggregate Regional Data

For MS-DRG 469 and 470, hospitals will be given information on average hospital spending in their region. The actual range and format has not been determined.

Timing of Baseline Data

Prior to the start of CJR, April 1, 2016, CMS will supply hospitals with 3 years of previous data.

Frequency of Claims Data Updates

CMS will make available the data upon a single initial request, rather than multiple periodic requests and updated data will be available no less frequently than once a month.

The Role of HIPAA

Despite the complexities of HIPAA, CMS has ruled that hospitals can share protected health information (PHI) with covered entities as long as that covered entity has a relationship with the patient. It is covered in that the hospital is using it for operations. Reasonable efforts must be used to limit the PHI to the minimum necessary. CMS will only be providing data to hospitals and will not provide it to collaborators or hospitals not in CJR. CMS has not decided whether to allow beneficiaries to opt-out of the CJR aspect of shared data.

Monitoring Beneficiary Protection

CMS is worried about increased steering of patients to lower cost, lower quality alternatives. While they think current safeguards are adequate, they want to increase them.

The CMS position is that hospitals can recommend other providers as long as they do not violate current laws and regulations. They must state to beneficiaries that these recommendations are not constrained.

Beneficiaries must be notified in many ways:

- Hospitals must make all notifications- descriptions of the CJR program and transparency with collaborators at the time of admission.
- General notice of the existence of the model
- Beneficiary rights
- Collaborators must also notify beneficiaries of their relationship separately and prior to the service being rendered
- Physicians must make all notifications at the time of the decision to proceed to surgery
- For PAC providers, hospitals must notify patients of all Medicare providers in the area but can identify those that are preferred.
- Hospitals must furnish the recently published list of all SNFs that qualify for a waiver of the 3-day rule

Monitoring for Access to Care

CMS will monitor for overutilization and underutilization of care. They will also monitor for differential increases or decreases reflecting shifting complex cases to other locations. In addition to penalties under existing law, hospitals can lose their reconciliation payments if this happens.

Monitoring for Quality of Care

While CMS believes that current professionalism and peer review is adequate, it reserves its right to review claims and to use QIO to assess for quality issues.

Additionally, to prevent directing patients to specific providers that would prevent choice to beneficiaries (which can be a quality issue), hospitals must provide a list of post-acute care providers as well as those that are collaborating. Collaborators must provide notice to the beneficiary that they are in a sharing agreement with the CJR hospital.

Monitoring for Delay of Care

To prevent postponing certain services until the end of the bundle, certain post-episode payments in the 30-day window after the episode will be counted and adjusted to the total episode.

Research Questions

CMS is overall interested in:
- Reduction in payments
- Decreases in utilization
- Outcomes/Quality
- Referral patterns and market impact
- Unintended consequences
- Potential to extrapolate results
- Explanations for variation of impact

Regulatory Impact Analysis

Under law, all regulations that can have greater than $100 million impact must have a regulatory impact analysis. CMS has done this.

The impact statement is in line with the rest of the ruling as CMS believes coordination of care will be improved, outcomes will be equal or better, and a significant amount of money will be saved.

CMS estimates that it will save 343 million dollars from 2016-2020.

Alphabetical List of Acronyms

µSA Micropolitan Statistical Area
ACE Acute Care Episode
ACO Accountable Care Organization
APM Alternative Payment Model
ASC Ambulatory Surgical Center
ASPE Assistant Secretary for Planning and Evaluation
BPCI Bundled Payments for Care Improvement
CAH Critical Access Hospital
CBSA Core-Based Statistical Area
CCN CMS Certification Number
CFR Code of Federal Regulations
CJR Comprehensive Care for Joint Replacement
CMHC Community Mental Health Center
CMI Case Mix Index
CMMI Center for Medicare and Medicaid Innovation CMP Civil Monetary Penalty
CMS Centers for Medicare & Medicaid Services
CoPs Conditions of Participation
CPCi Comprehensive Primary Care Initiative
CPT Current Procedural Terminology
CSA Combined Statistical Area
DME Durable Medical Equipment
DMEPOS Durable Medical Equipment, Prosthetics, Orthotics, and Supplies
eCQM Electronic Clinical Quality Measures
EFT Electronic funds transfer
ESRD End-Stage Renal Disease
FFS Fee-for-service
GAAP Generally Accepted Accounting Principles
GEM General Equivalence Mapping
GPCI Geographic Practice Cost Index
HAC Hospital-Acquired Condition
HACRP Hospital-Acquired Condition Reduction Program
HCAHPS Hospital Consumer Assessment of Healthcare Providers and Systems
HCC Hierarchical Condition Category
HCPCS Healthcare Common Procedure Coding System
HHA Home health agency
HHPPS Home Health Prospective Payment System
HHRG Home Health Resource Group
HHVBP Home Health Value-Based Purchasing
HIT Health Information Technology
HIQR Hospital Inpatient Quality Reporting
HLMR HCAHPS Linear Mean Roll Up
HOOS Hip Dysfunction and Osteoarthritis Outcome Score
HOPD Hospital outpatient department
HRR Hospital Referral Region

HRRP Hospital Readmissions Reductions Program
HVBP Hospital Value Based Purchasing Program
ICD–9–CM International Classification of Diseases, 9th Revision, Clinical Modification
ICD–10–CM International Classification of Diseases, 10th Revision, Clinical Modification
IPPS Inpatient Prospective Payment System
IPF Inpatient psychiatric facility
IRF Inpatient rehabilitation facility
KOOS Knee Injury and Osteoarthritis Outcome Score
LEJR Lower extremity joint replacement
LOS Length of stay
LTCH Long term care hospital
LUPA Low Utilization Payment Adjustment
MAC Medicare Administrative Contractor
MACRA Medicare Access and Chip Reauthorization Act of 2015
MAPCP Multi-Payer Advanced Primary Care Practice model
MCC Major Complications or Comorbidities
MCCM Medicare Care Choices Model
MDH Medicare-Dependent Hospital
MedPAC Medicare Payment Advisory Commission
MIPS Merit-based Incentive Payment System
MP Malpractice
MPFS Medicare Physician Fee Schedule
MSA Metropolitan Statistical Area
MS–DRG Medical Severity Diagnosis Related Group
NPI National Provider Identifier
NPP Nonphysician Practitioner
NPRA Net Payment Reconciliation Amount
NQF National Quality Forum
OCM Oncology Care Model
OPPS Outpatient Prospective Payment System
PAC Post-Acute Care
PBPM Per Beneficiary Per Month
PE Practice Expense
PGP Physician Group Practice
PHA Partial hip arthroplasty
PPS Prospective Payment System
PRO Patient-Reported Outcome
PROMIS Patient-Reported Outcomes Measurement Information Systems
PRO–PM Patient-Reported Outcome Performance Measure
QIO Quality Improvement Organization
RAC Recovery Audit Contractor
RRC Rural Referral Center
RSCR Risk-Standardized Complication Rate
RSRR Risk-Standardized Readmission Rate

RVU Relative Value Unit
SCH Sole Community Hospital
SNF Skilled nursing facility
THA Total hip arthroplasty
TIN Taxpayer identification number
TKA Total knee arthroplasty
TP Target price
VR–12 Veterans Rand 12 Item Health Survey

PART 510-COMPREHENSIVE CARE FOR JOINT REPLACEMENT MODEL

Sec.

Authority: Secs. 1102, 1115A, and 1871 of the Social Security Act (42 U.S.C. 1302, 1315(a), and 1395hh).

SUbpart A-General Provisions

§510.1 Baals andacope.

(a) *Basis.* This part implements the test of the Comprehensive Care for Joint Replacement model under section 1115A of the Act. Except as specifically noted in this part, the regulations under this part must not be construed to affect the payment, coverage, program integrity, or other requirements (such as those in parts 412 and 482 of this chapter) that apply to pro viders and suppliers under this chapter.

(b} *Scope.* This part sets forth the following:

(1) The participants in the Comprehensive Care for Joint Replacement model.

(2) The episodes being tested in the model.

(3) The methodology for pricing and payment under the model.

(4) Quality performance standards and quality reporting requirements.

(5) Safeguards to ensure preservation of beneficiary choice and beneficiary notification.

§510.2 Definitions.

For the purposes of this part, the following definitions are applicable unless otherwise stated:

AGO stands for accountable care organization.

Actual episode payment means the sum of Medicare claims payments for items and services that are included in the episode in accordance with §510.200(b), excluding the items and services described in §510.200(d).

Alignment payment means a payment from a CJR collaborator to a participant hospital under a sharing arrangement, for only the purpose of sharing the participant hospital's responsibility for repayments to Medicare.

Anchor hospitalization means the initial hospital stay upon admission for a lower extremity joint replacement.

BPCI stands for the Bundled Payment for Care Improvement initiative.

CEC stands for Comprehensive ESRD Care Initiative.

CCN stands for CMS certification number.

CJR collaborator means one of the following Medicare.enrolled persons or entities that enters into a sharing arrangement:

　(1) Skilled nursing facility (SNF).

　(2) Home health agency (HHA).

　(3) Long-term care hospital (LTCH).

　(4) Inpatient rehabilitation facility (IRF).

　(5) Physician.

　(6) NonJ?hysician practitioner.

　(7) Provider or supplier of outpatient therapy services.

　(8) Physician group practice (PGP).

CJR reconciliation report means the report prepared after each reconciliation that CMS provides to each participant hospital notifying the participant hospital of the outcome of the reconciliation.

Collaborator agreement means a written, signed agreement between a CJR collaborator and a participant hospital that meets the requirements of §510.500(c).

Composite quality score means a score computed for each participant hospital to summarize the hospital's level of quality performance and improvement on specified quality measures as described in §510.315.

Core-based statistical area (CBSA) means a statistical geographic entity consisting of the county or counties associated with at least one core (urbanized area or urban cluster) of at least 10,000 population, plus adjacent counties having a high degree of social and economic integration with the core as measured through commuting ties with the counties containing the core.

Critical access hospital {CAH) means a hospital designated under subpart F of part 485 of this chapter.

Distribution arrangement means a financial arrangement between a PGP that is a CJR collaborator and a practice collaboration agent in which the PGP distributes some or all of a gainsharing payment that it received from a participant hospital.

Distribution payment means a payment made by a PGP that is a CJR collaborator to a practice collaboration agent under a distribution arrangement.

DME stands for durable medical equipment.

EFT stands for electronic funds transfer.

Episode of care {or Episode) means all Medicare Part A and B items and services described in §510.200(b) (and excluding the items and services described in §510.200(d)) that are furnished to a beneficiary described in §510.205 during the time period that begins with the beneficiary's admission to an anchor hospitalization and ends on the 90th day after the date of discharge from the anchor hospitalization, with the day of discharge itself being counted as the first day of the 90-day post-discharge period.

Episode target price means the amount determined in accordance with §510.300 and applied to an episode in determining a net payment reconciliation amount.

ESRD stands for end stage renal disease.

Gainsharing payment means a payment from a participant hospital to a CJR collaborator, under a sharing arrangement, composed of only reconciliation payments or internal cost savings or both.

HHA stands for home health agency.

HCAHPS stands for Hospital Consumer Assessment of Healthcare Providers and Systems.

HCPCS stands for CMS Common Procedure Coding System.

Historical episode payment means the most recent 3 years of expenditures for an episode in a given participant hospital.

ICD-CM stands for International Classification of Diseases, Clinical Modification.

Inpatient prospective payment systems (IPPS) means the payment systems for subsection (d) hospitals as defined in section 1886(d)(1)(B) of the Act.

Internal cost savings means the measurable, actual, and verifiable cost savings realized by the participant hospital resulting from care redesign undertaken by the participant hospital in connection with providing items and services to beneficiaries within specific CJR episodes of care. Internal cost savings does not include savings realized by any individual or entity that is not the participant hospital.

IPF stands for inpatient psychiatric facility.

!PPS hospital {or hospital) means a provider subject to the prospective payment system specified in §412.1(a)(1) of this chapter.

IRF stands for inpatient rehabilitation facility.

Lawer-extremity joint replacement {LE/R) means any procedure that is within MS-DRG 469 or 470, including lower.extremity joint replacement

procedures or reattachment of a lower extremity.

LTCH stands for long-term care hospital.

Medicare severity diagnosis-related group (MS-DRG} means, for the purposes of this model, the classification of inpatient hospital discharges updated in accordance with §412.10 of this chapter.

Medicare-dependent, small rural hospital {MDH) means a specific type of hospital that meets the classification criteria specified under §412.108 of this chapter.

Member of the PGP or *PGP member* means a physician, nonphysician practitioner, or therapist who is an owner or employee of the PGP and who has reassigned to the PGP his or her right to receive Medicare payment.

Metropolitan Statistical Area (MSA} means a core-based statistical area associated with at least one urbanized area that has a population of at least 50,000.

Net payment reconciliation amount (NPRA} means the amount determined in accordance with § 510.305(e).

Nonphysician practitioner means (except for purposes of subpart G of this part) one of the following:

　(1) A physician assistant who satisfies the qualifications set forth at §410.74(a)(2)(i) and (ii) of this chapter.

　(2) A nurse practitioner who satisfies the qualifications set forth at §410.75(b) of this chapter.

　(3) A clinical nurse specialist who satisfies the qualifications set forth at §410.76(b) of this chapter.

　(4) A certified registered nurse anesthetist (as defined at §410.69(bl).

　(5) A clinical social worker (as defined at §410.73(al).

　(6) A registered dietician or nutrition professional (as defined at §410.134).

NPI stands for National Provider Identifier.

OIG stands for the Department of Health and Human Services Office of the Inspector General.

PAC stands for post-acute care.

Participant hospital means an IPPS hospital (other than those hospitals specifically excepted under §510.lOO(b)) with a CCN primary address in one of the geographic areas selected for participation in the CJR model in accordance with §510.105, as of the date of selection or any time thereafter during any performance period.

PBPM stands for per-beneficiary-per-month.

Performance year means one of the years in which the CJR model is being tested. Performance years for the model correlate to calendar years with the exception of performance year 1, which is April 1, 2016 through December 31, 2016.

PGP stands for physician group practice.

Physician has the meaning set forth in section 1861(r) of the Act.

Post-episode spending amount means the sum of Medicare Parts A and B payments for items and services that are furnished to a beneficiary within 30 days after the end of the beneficiary's episode.

Practice collaboration agent means a PGP member who has entered into a distribution arrangement with the same PGP of which he or she is a member and who has not entered into a collaborator agreement with a participant hospital.

Provider of outpatient therapy seivices means a provider or supplier furnishing one or more of the following:

(1) Outpatient physical therapy services as defined in §410.60 of this chapter.

(2) Outpatient occupational therapy services as defined in §410.59 of this chapter.

(3) Outpatient speech-language pathology services as defined in §410.62 of this chapter.

Quality improvement points are points that CMS adds to a participant hospital's composite quality score for a measure if the hospital's performance percentile on an individual quality measure increases from the previous performance year by at least 3 deciles on the performance percentile scale.

Quality performance points are points that CMS adds to a participant hospital's composite quality score for a measure based on the performance percentile scale and for successful data submission of patient-reported outcomes.

Reconciliation payment means a payment made by CMS to a CJR participant hospital as determined in accordance with §510.305(1').

Region means one of the nine U.S. census divisions, as defined by the U.S. Census Bureau.

Repayment amount means the amount owed by a participant hospital to CMS, as reflected on a reconciliation report

Rural hospital means an IPPS hospital that meets one of the following definitions:

[1) Is located in a rural area as defined under §412.64 of this chapter.

(2) Is located in a rural census tract defined under §412.103(a)(1) of this chapter.

(3) Has reclassified as a rural hospital under §412.103 of this chapter.

Rural referral center (RRC) has the same meaning given this term under §412.96 of this chapter.

Sharing armngement means a financial arrangement between a participant hospital and a CJR collaborator for the sole purpose of making gainsharing payments or alignment payments under the CJR model.

Sole community hospital (SCH) means a hospital that meets the classification criteria specified in §412.92 of this chapter.

SNF stands for skilled nursing facility.

Therapist means one of the following as defined at §484.4:

(1) Physical therapist.

(2) Occupational therapist.

(3) Speech-language pathologist.

TKAITHA stands for total knee arthroplasty/total hip arthroplasty.

TIN stands for taxpayer identification number.

Subpart B-Comprehenaive care for Joint Replacement Program Participants

§510,100   Epleodea being INted.

(a) *Initiation of an episode.* An episode is initiated when a participant hospital admits a Medicare beneficiary described in §510.205 for an anchor hospitalization.

(b) *Exclusions.* A hospital is excluded from being a participant hospital, but only so long as any of the following conditions apply:

(1) The hospital is an episode initiator for an LEJR episode in the risk-bearing period of Models 2 or 4 of BPCI.

(2) The hospital is participating in Model 1 of BPCI.

(3) These exclusions cease to apply as of the date that the hospital no longer meets any of the conditions specified in this paragraph.

§510.105   le lll'Na.

[a] *General.* The geographic areas for inclusion in the CJR model are obtained based on a stratified random sampling of certain MSAs in the United States. All counties within each of the selected MSAs are selected for inclusion in the CJR model.

(b) *Stratification criteria.* Geographic areas in the United States are stratified according to the characteristics that CMS determines are necessary to ensure that the model is tested on a broad range of different types of hospitals that may face different obstacles and incentives for improving quality and controlling costs.

(c) *Exclusions.* CMS excludes from the selection of geographic areas MSAs that met the following criteria:

(1) Had fewer than 400 episodes between July 1, 2013 and June 30, 2014.

(2) Had fewer than 400 non-Model 1, 2, or 4 BPCI episodes as of October 1, 2015.

(3) Failed either or both of the following rules regarding participation in BPCI:

(i) More than 50 percent of eligible episodes initiated in a BPCI Model 2 or 4 initiating hospital.

[ii) More than 50 percent of eligible episodes that included SNF or HHA services, where the SNF or HHA services were furnished by a BPCI Model 3 initiating HHA or SNF.

{4) For MSAs including both Maryland and non-Maryland counties, more than 50 percent of eligible episodes were initiated at a Maryland hospital.

Subpart C-Scope of Episodee

§510.200   Time periods, included and excluckld Hrvlcff, and attribution.

(a) *Time periods.* All episodes must begin on or after April 1, 2016 and end on or before December 31, 2020.

(b) *Included services.* All Medicare Parts A and B items and services are included in the episode, except as specified in paragraph (d) of this section. These services include, but are not limited to, the following:

(1) Physicians' services.

(2) Inpatient hospital services (including hospital readmissions}.

(3) IPF services.

(4) LTCH services.

(5) JRF services.

(6) SNF services.

(1) HHA services.

(8) Hospital outpatient services.

(9) Outpatient therapy services.

(10) Clinical laboratory services.

[ll) DME.

(12) Part B drugs and biologicals.

(13) Hospice services.

(14) PBPM payments under models tested under section 1115A of the Act.

(c) *Episode attribution.* All items and services included in the episode are attributed to the participant hospital at which the anchor hospitalization occurs.

(d) *Excluded services.* The following items, services, and payments are excluded from the episode:

(1) Hemophilia clotting factors provided in accordance with §412.115 of this chapter.

(2) New technology add-on payments, as defined in part 412, subpart F of this chapter.

(3) Transitional pass-through payments for medical devices as defined in §419.66 of this chapter.

(4) Items and services unrelated to the anchor hospitalization, as determined by CMS. Excluded services include, but are not limited to, the following:

45

(i) Inpatient hospital admissions for MS-DRGs that group to the following categories of diagnoses:

(Al Oncology.

(Bl Trauma medical.

(Cl Chronic disease surgical, such as prostatectomy.

(D) Acute disease surgical, such as appendectomy.

(ii) Medicare Part B services, as identified by the principal ICD-CM diagnosis code on the claim (based on the ICD-CM version in use during the performance year) that group to the following categories of diagnoses:

(A) Acute disease diagnoses, such as severe head injury.

(B) Certain chronic disease diagnoses. as specified by CMS on a diagnosis-by-diagnosis basis depending on whether the condition was likely to have been affected by the LEJR procedure and recovery period or whether substantial services were likely to be provided for the chronic condition during the episode. Such chronic disease diagnoses are posted on the CMS Web site and may be revised in accordance with paragraph (el of this section.

(iii) Certain PBPM payments under models tested under section 1115A of the Act. PBPM model payments that CMS determines to be primarily used for care coordination or care management services for clinical conditions in excluded categories of diagnoses, as described in this paragraph.

(Al The list of excluded PBPM payments is posted on the CMS Web site and are revised in accordance with paragraph (el of this section.

(Bl Notwithstanding the foregoing, all PBPM model payments funded from CMS' Innovation Center appropriation are excluded from the episode.

(5) Certain incentive programs and add on payments under existing Medicare payment systems in accordance with §510.300(b)(6) of this chapter.

(6) Payments for otherwise included items and services in excess of 2 standard deviations above the mean regional episode payment in accordance with §510.300(b)(5) of this chapter.

(el *Updating the lists of excluded services.* (1) The list of excluded MS-DRGs, ICD-CM diagnosis codes, and CMS model PBPM payments are posted on the CMS Web site.

(2) On an annual basis, or more frequently as needed, CMS updates the list of excluded services to reflect annual coding changes or other issues brought to CMS's attention.

(3) CMS applies the following standards when revising the list of

excluded services for reasons other than to reflect annual coding changes:

(i) Items or services that are directly related to the LEJR procedure or the quality or safety of LEJR care would be included in the episode.

(ii) Items or services for chronic conditions that may be affected by the LEJR procedure or post-surgical care would be related and included in the episode.

(iii) Items and services for chronic conditions that are generally not affected by the LEJR procedure or post-surgical care would be excluded from the episode.

(iv) Items and services for acute clinical conditions not arising from existing, episode-related chronic clinical conditions or complications of LEJR surgery would be excluded from the episode.

(v) PBPM payments under CMS models determined to be primarily used for care coordination or care management services for clinical conditions in excluded categories of diagnoses, as described in §510.200(d), would be excluded from the episode.

(4) CMS posts the following to the CMS Web site:

(i) Potential revisions to the exclusion to allow for public comment; and

(ii) An updated exclusions list after consideration of public comment.

§510.205 Beneficiary Inclualon criteria.

(a) Episodes tested in the CJR model include only those in which care is furnished to beneficiaries who meet all of the following criteria upon admission to the anchor hospitalization:

(1) Are enrolled in Medicare Parts A and Part B.

(2) Eligibility for Medicare is not on the basis of end stage renal disease, as described in §406.13 of this chapter.

(3) Are not enrolled in any managed care plan (for example, Medicare Advantage, health care prepayment plans, or cost-based health maintenance organizations).

(4) Are not covered under a United Mine Workers of America health care plan.

(5) Have Medicare as their primary payer.

(bl Ifat any time during the episode a beneficiary no longer meets all of the criteria in this section, the episode is canceled in accordance with §510.210(b).

§510.21 O OatannlnaUon of the episode.

(al *General.* The episode begins with the admission of a Medicare beneficiary described in §510.205 to a participant hospital for an anchor hospitalization and ends on the 90th day after the date

of discharge, with the day of discharge itself being counted as the first day in the 90-day post-discharge period.

(b) *Cancellation of an episode.* The episode is canceled and is not included in the determination of NPRA as specified in §510.305 if the beneficiary does any of the following during the episode:

(l) Ceases to meet any criterion listed in §510.205.

(2) Is readmitted to any participant hospital for another anchor hospitalization.

(3) Initiates an LEJR episode under BPCI.

(4) Dies.

Subpart D-Prfclng and Payment

§510.300 Oetannlnauon of episode target prices.

(a) *General.* CMS establishes episode target prices for participant hospitals for each performance year of the model as specified in this section. Episode target prices are established according to the following:

(1) MS-DRG assigned at discharge for anchor hospitalization and presence of hip fracture diagnosis for anchor hospitalization-

(i) MS-DRG 469 with hip fracture;

(ii) MS-DRG 469 without hip fracture;

(iii) MS-DRG 470 with hip fracture; or

(iv) MS-DRG 470 without hip fracture.

(2) *Applicable time period for performance* year *episode target prices.* Episode target prices are updated to account for Medicare payment updates no less than 2 times per year, for updated episode target prices effective October 1 and January 1, and at other intervals if necessary.

(3) *Episodes that straddle performance years* or *payment updates.* The episode target price that applies to the type of episode as of the date of admission for the anchor hospitalization is the episode target price that applies to the episode.

(4) Adjustments for quality performance, as specified in §510.305(g).

(5) *Identifying episodes with hip fracture.* CMS develops a list of ICD-CM hip fracture diagnosis codes that, when reported in the principal diagnosis code files on the claim for the anchor hospitalization, represent a bone fracture for which a hip replacement procedure, either a partial hip arthroplasty or a total hip arthroplasty, could be the primary surgical treatment. The list of ICD-CM hip fracture diagnosis codes used to identify hip fracture episodes is posted on the CMS Web site.

(i) On an annual basis, or more frequently as needed, CMS updates the list of ICD-CM hip fracture diagnosis codes to reflect coding changes or other issues brought to CMS' attention.

(ii) CMS applies the following standards when revising the list of ICD-CM hip fracture diagnosis codes.

(Al The ICD-CM diagnosis code is sufficiently specific that it represents a bone fracture for which a physician could determine that a hip replacement procedure, either a PHA or a THA, could be the primary surgical treatment.

(Bl The ICD-CM diagnosis code is the primary reason (that is, principal diagnosis code) for the anchor hosr.italization.

(iii) CMS posts the following to the CMS Web site:

(A) Potential ICD-CM hip fracture diagnosis codes for public comment; and

(Bl A final ICD-CM hip fracture diagnosis code list after consideration of public comment.

(bl *Episode target price.* (1)CMS calculates episode target prices based on a blend of each participant hospital's hospital-specific and regional episode expenditures. The region corresponds to the U.S. Census Division associated with the primary address of the CCN of the participant hospital and the regional component is based on all hospitals in said region, except as follows. In cases where an MSA selected for participation in CJR spans more than one U.S. Census Division, the entire MSA will be grouped into the U.S. Census Division where the largest city by population in the MSA is located for target price and reconciliation calculations. The calendar years used for historical expenditure calculations are as follows:

(i) Episodes beginning in 2012 through 2014 for performance years 1 and 2.

(ii) Episodes beginning in 2014 through 2016 for performance years 3 and 4.

(iii) Episodes beginning in 2016 through 2018 for performance year 5.

(2) Specifically, the blend consists of the following:

(i) Two-thirds of the participant hospital's own historical episode payments and one-third of the regional historical episode payments for performance years 1and 2.

(ii) One-third of the hospital's own historical episode payments and two-thirds of the regional historical episode payments for performance year 3.

(iii) Regional historical episode payments for performance years 4 and 5.

(3) *Exception for low-volume hospitals.* Episode target prices for participant hospitals with fewer than 20 CJR episodes in total across the 3 historical years of data used to calculate the episode target price are based on 100 percent regional historical episode payments.

(4) *Exception for recently merged or split hospitals.* Hospital-specific historical episode payments for participant hospitals that have undergone a merger, consolidation, spin off or other reorganization that results in a new hospital entity without 3 full years of historical claims data are determined using the historical episode payments attributed to their predecessor(s).

(5) *Exception for high episode spending.* Episode payments are capped at 2 standard deviations above the mean regional episode payment for both the hospital-specific and regional comronents of the target price.

(6 *Exclusion of incentive programs and add-on payments under existing Medicare payment systems.* Certain incentive programs and add-on payments are excluded from historical episode payments by using the CMS Price (Payment) Standardization Detailed Methodology used for the Medicare spending per beneficiary measure in the Hospital Value-Based Purchasing Program.

(7) *Communication of episode target prices.* CMS communicates episode target prices to participant hospitals before the performance period in which they apply.

(cl *Discount factor.* A participant hospital's episode target prices incorporate applicable discount factors to reflect Medicare's portion of reduced expenditures from the CJR model as described in this section.

(1) *Discount factor for reconciliation payments.* The applicable discount factor for reconciliation payments in all performance years is 3.0 percent.

(2) *Discount factors for repayment amounts.* The applicable discount factor for repayment amounts are-

(i) Not applicable in performance year 1, as the requirement for hospital repayment under the CJR model is waived in performance year l;

(ii) In performance years 2 and 3, 2.0 percent; and

(3) *Discount factors affected by the quality incentive payment and composite performance years.* In all performance years, the discount factor may be affected by the quality incentive payment and composite quality score as provided in §510.315 to create a different effective discount factor used for calculating reconciliation payments and repayment amounts.

(d) *Data sharing.* (1)CMS makes available to participant hospitals, through the most appropriate means, data that CMS determines may be useful to participant hospitals to do the following:

(i) Determine appropriate ways to increase the coordination of care.

(ii) Improve quality.

(iii) Enhance efficiencies in the delivery of care.

(iv) Otherwise achieve the goals of the CJR model described in this section.

(2) *Beneficiary-identifiable data.* (i) CMS makes beneficiary-identifiable data available to a participant hospital in accordance with applicable privacy laws and only in response to the hospital's request for such data for a beneficiary who has been furnished a billable service by the participant hospital corresponding to the episode definitions for CJR.

(ii) The minimum data necessary to achieve the goals of the CJR model, as determined by CMS, may be provided under this section for a participant hospital's baseline period and no less frequently than on a quarterly basis throughout the hospital's participation in the CJR model.

§510.305 Detennlnaaon of the NPRA and reconclllaaon process.

(a) *Generol.* Providers and suppliers furnishing items and services included in the episode bill for such items and services in accordance with existing rules and as if this part were not in effect.

(b) *Reconciliation.* CMS uses a series of reconciliation processes, which CMS performs as described in paragraphs (d) and (f) of this section after the end of each performance year, to establish final payment amounts to participant hospitals for CJR episodes for a given performance year. Following the end of each performance year, CMS determines actual episode payments for each episode for the performance year (other than episodes that have been canceled in accordance with §510.210(b)) and determines the amount of a reconciliation payment or repayment amount.

(cl *Data used.* CMS uses the most recent claims data available to perform each reconciliation calculation.

(d) *Annual reconciliation.* (1) Beginning 2 months after the end of each performance year, CMS performs a reconciliation calculation to establish an NPRA for each participant hospital.

(2) **CMS-**

(i) Calculates the NPRA for each participant hospital in accordance with paragraph (el of this section including the adjustments provided for in paragraph (e)(l)(iv) of this section; and

(ii) Assesses whether hospitals meet specified quality requirements under §510.315.

(e) *Calculation of the NPRA.* By comparing the episode target prices described in §510.300 and the participant hospital's actual episode spending for the performance year and applying the adjustments in paragraph (e)(1)(v) of this section, CMS establishes an NPRA for each participant hospital for each performance year.

(1) *Initial calculation.* In calculating the NPRA for each participant hospital for each performance year, CMS does the followin:

(i) Determines actual episode payments for each episode included in the performance year (other than episodes that have been canceled in accordance with §510.210(b)) using claims data that is available 2 months after the end of the performance year. Actual episode payments are capped at the amount determined in accordance with §510.300(b)(5) for the performance year.

(ii) Multiplies each episode target price, after applying any reduction to the discount percentage as provided in §510.315(f) by the number of episodes included in the performance year (other than episodes that have been canceled in accordance with §510.210(b)) to which that episode target price applies.

(iii) Aggregates the amounts computed in paragraph (e)(1)(ii) of this section for all episodes included in the performance year (other than episodes that have been canceled in accordance with §510.210(b)).

(iv) Subtracts the amount determined under paragraph (e)(1)(i) of this section from the amount determined under paragraph (e)(1)(iii) of this section.

(v) Makes the following adjustments:

(A) *Increases in post-episode spending.* If the average post-episode Medicare Parts A and B spending for a participant hospital in any given performance year is greater than 3 standard deviations above the regional average post-episode spending for the same performance year, then the spending amount exceeding three standard deviations above the regional average post-episode spending for the same performance year is applied to the NPRA.

(B) *Limitation on loss.* Except as provided in paragraph (e)(1)(v)(D) of this section, the total amount any participant hospital is responsible for repaying to Medicare for a performance year cannot exceed the following:

(1) For performance year 2 only, 5 percent of the amount calculated in paragraph (e)(1)(iii) of this section for the performance year.

(2) For performance year 3, 10 percent of the amount calculated in paragraph (e)(1)(iii) of this section for the performance year.

(3) For performance years 4, and 5, 20 percent of the amount calculated in paragraph (e)(1)(iii) of this section for the performance year.

(4) As provided in paragraph (h)(6)(i) of this section, the subsequent reconciliation calculation reassesses the limitation on loss for a given performance year by applying the limitations on loss to the aggregate of the 2 reconciliation calculations.

(C) *Limitation on gain.* The total amount of any reconciliation payment made to a participant hospital for a performance year cannot exceed the following:

(1) For performance years 1 and 2, 5 percent of the amount calculated in paragraph (e)(1)(iii) of this section for the performance year.

(2) For performance year 3, 10 percent of the amount calculated in paragraph (e)(1)(iii) of this section for the performance year.

(3) For performance years 4, and 5, 20 percent of the amount calculated in paragraph (e)(1)(iii) of this section for the performance year.

(4) As provided in paragraph (h)(6)(i) of this section, the subsequent reconciliation calculation reassesses the limitation on gain for a given performance year by applying the limitation on gain limits to the aggregate of the two reconciliation calculations.

(D) *Financial loss limits for rural hospitals, SCHs, MDHs, and RRCs.* If a participant hospital is a rural hospital, SCH, MDH or RRC, then for performance year 2, the total repayment amount for which the participant hospital is responsible cannot exceed 3 percent of the amount calculated in paragraph (e)(1)(iii) of this section. For performance years 3 through 5, the total repayment amount cannot exceed 5 percent of the amount calculated in paragraph (e)(1)(iii) of this section.

(f) *Determination of reconciliation or repayment amount*- (1) *Determination of the reconciliation or repayment amount.* (i) Subject to paragraph (f)(1)(iii) of this section, for performance year 1, the reconciliation payment (if any) is equal to the NPRA.

(ii) Subject to paragraph (f)(1)(iii) of this section, for performance years 2 through 5, results from the subsequent reconciliation calculation for a prior year's reconciliation, as described in paragraph (h)(6)(i) of this section, are applied to the current year's NPRA in order to determine the reconciliation or repayment amount.

(iii) The reconciliation or repayment amount may be adjusted as provided in §510.410(b)(5).

(2) *Reconciliation payment.* If the amount described in paragraph (f)(1) of this section is positive and the composite quality score described in §510.315 is acceptable (defined as greater than or equal to 4.00), good (defined as greater than or equal to 6.0 and less than or equal to 13.2), or excellent (defined as greater than 13.2), Medicare pays the participant hospital a reconciliation payment in an amount equal to the amount described in paragraph (f)(1) of this section.

(3) *Repayment amount.* If the amount described in paragraph (f)(1) of this section is negative, the participant hospital pays to Medicare an amount equal to the amount described in paragraph (f)(1) of this section, in accordance with §405.371 of this chapter. CMS waives this requirement for performance year 1.

(g) *Determination of eligibility for reconciliation based on quality.* (1) CMS assesses each participant hospital's performance on quality metrics, as described in §510.315, to determine whether the participant hospital is eligible to receive a reconciliation payment for a performance year.

(2) If the hospital's composite quality score described in §510.315 is acceptable (defined as greater than or equal to 4.00), good (defined as greater than or equal to 6.0 and less than or equal to 13.2), or excellent (defined as greater than 13.2), and the hospital is determined to have a positive NPRA under §510.305(e)), the hospital is eligible for a reconciliation payment.

(3) If the hospital's composite quality score described in §510.315 is below acceptable, defined as less than 4.00 for a performance year, the hospital is not eligible for a reconciliation payment.

(4) If the hospital is found to be engaged in an inappropriate and systemic under delivery of care, the quality of the care provided must be considered to be seriously compromised and the hospital must be ineligible to receive or retain a reconciliation payment for any period in which such under delivery of care was found to occur.

(h) *Reconciliation report.* CMS issues each participant hospital a CJR reconciliation report for the performance year. Each CJR reconciliation report contains the following:

(1) Information on the participant hospital's composite quality score described in §510.315.

(2) The total actual episode payments for the participant hospital.

(3) The NPRA.

(4) Whether the participant hospital is eligible for a reconciliation payment or must make a repayment to Medicare.

(5) The NPRA and subsequent reconciliation calculation amount for the previous performance year, as applicable.

(6) The reconciliation payment or repayment amount.

(i) *Subsequent reconciliotion calculation.* (Al Fourteen months after the end of each performance year, CMS performs an additional calculation, using claims data available at that time, to account for final claims run-out and any additional overlap between the CJR model and other CMS models and programs as described in paragraph (h)(6)(i)(B) of this section.

(Bl The subsequent reconciliation calculation accounts for cases in which a portion of the CJR discount percentage is paid out to an ACO as shared savings by reducing the reconciliation payment amount for a CJR hospital, if available, by the amount of the discount percentage paid out to the ACO as shared savings. This adjustment is only made when the participant hospital is a participant or provider/supplier in the ACO and the beneficiary in the CJR episode is assigned to one of the following ACO models or program:

(1) The Pioneer ACO model.

(2) The Medicare Shared Savings **Pro.**

(3) The Next Generation ACO model.

(4) The Comprehensive ESRD Care Initiative.

(Cl The additional calculation occurs concurrently with the reconciliation process for the most recent performance year. Ifthe result of the subsequent calculation is different than zero, CMS applies the stop-loss and stop-gain limits in paragraph (el of this section to the calculations in aggregate for that performance year (the initial reconciliation and the subsequent calculation) to ensure the amount does not exceed the stop-loss or stop-gain limits. CMS then applies the subsequent calculation amount to the NPRA for the most recent performance year in order to determine the reconciliation amount or repayment amount for the most recent performance year. Because hospitals will not have financial repayment responsibility for performance year 1, for the performance year 2 reconciliation report only, the subsequent calculation amount (for performance year 1) is applied to the performance year 1 NPRA to ensure that the combined amount is not less than O. Ifthe combined performance year 1 NPRA and subsequent calculation for performance year 1 is less than 0, the

subsequent calculation amount would be capped at the value that would result in a net amount of O for the combined performance year 1NPRA and subsequent calculation.

§510.310 Appeals proceq.

(a) *Notice of calculation error (first level of appeal).* Subject to the limitations on review in subpart d of this part, if a participant hospital wishes to dispute the calculation that involves a matter related to payment, reconciliation amounts, repayment amounts, or determinations associated with quality measures affecting payment, the hospital is required to provide written notice of the error, in a form and manner specified by CMS.

(1) Unless the participant liospital provides such notice, the CJR reconciliation report is deemed final 45 calendar days after it is issued.

(2) IfCMS receives a timely notice of a calculation error, CMS responds in writing within 30 calendar days to either confirm that there was an error in the calculation or verify that the calculation is correct, although CMS reserves the right to an extension upon written notice to the participant hospital.

(3) If a participant hospital does not submit timely notice of a calculation error in accordance with the timelines and processes specified by CMS, then CMS deems final the CJR reconciliation report and proceeds with the payment or repayment processes, as applicable.

(4) Only participant hospitals may use the dispute resolution process described in this art.

(b) *Dispute resolution process (second level of appeal).* (1) Ifthe participant hospital is dissatisfied with CMS's response to the notice of a calculation error, the participant hospital may request a reconsideration review in a form and manner as specified by CMS.

(2) The reconsideration review request must provide a detailed explanation of the basis for the dispute and include supporting documentation for the participant hospital's assertion that CMS or its representatives did not accurately calculate the NPRA, the reconciliation payment, or the repayment amount in accordance with §510.305.

(3) If CMS does not receive a request for reconsideration from the participant hospital within 10 calendar days of the issue date of CMS's response to the participant hospital's notice of calculation error, then CMS's response to the calculation error is deemed final and CMS proceeds with reconciliation payment or repayment processes, as applicable, as described in §510.305.

(4) A CMS reconsideration official notifies the participant hospital in writing within 15 calendar days of receiving the participant hospital's review request of the following:

(i) The date, time, and location of the review.

(ii) The issues in dispute.

(iii) The review procedures.

(iv) The procedures (including format and deadlines) for submission of evidence.

(5) The CMS reconsideration official takes all reasonable efforts to schedule the review to occur no later than 30 days after the date of receipt of the notification.

(6) The provisions at §425.804(bJ, (c), and (el of this chapter are applicable to reviews conducted in accordance with the reconsideration review process for **CJR**

(7) The CMS reconsideration official issues a written determination within 30 days of the review. The determination is final and binding.

(c) *Exception to the process.* Ifthe participant hospital contests a matter that does not involve an issue contained in, or a calculation which contributes to, a CJR reconciliation report, a notice of calculation error is not required. An exampie of such a matter is termination of the participant hospital from the model. In those instances, if CMS does not receive a request for reconsideration from the participant hospital within 10 calendar days of the notice of the initial determination, the initial determination is deemed final and CMS proceeds with action indicated in the initial determination.

(d) *Limitations* on *review.* In accordance with section 1115A(d)(2) of the Act, there is no administrative or judicial review under sections 1869 or 1878 of the Act or otherwise for the following:

(l) The selection of models for testing or expansion under section 1115A of the Act.

(2) The selection of organizations, sites, or participants to test those models selected.

(3) The elements, parameters, scope. and duration of such models for testing or dissemination.

(4) Determinations regarding budget neutrality under section 1115A(b)(3) of Act.

(5) The termination or modification of the design and implementation of a model under section 1115A(b)(3)(B) of Act.

(6) Decisions about expansion of the duration and scope of a model under section 1115A(c) of the Act, including the determination that a model is not

49

expected to meet criteria described in paragraph (d)(1) or (2) of this section.

§510.315 Cornpoelte quality scores for detennlnlng reconctllatton payment ellglblllty and quality Incentive payments.

(a) *General.* A participant hospital's eligibility for a reconciliation payment under §510.305(g), and the determination of quality incentive payments under paragraph (f) of this section, for a performance year depend on the hospital's composite quality score (including any quality performance points and quality improvement points earned) for that performance year.

(b) *Composite quality score.* CMS calculates a composite quality score for each participant hospital for each performance year, which equals the sum of the following:

(1) The hospital's quality performance points for the hospital-level risk-standardized complication rate following elective primary total hip arthroplasty and/or total knee arthroplasty measure (NQF #1550) described in §510.400(a)(1). This measure is weighted at 50 percent of the composite quality score.

(2) The hospital's quality performance points for the Hospital Consumer Assessment of Healthcare Providers and Systems Survey measure (NQF #0166) described in §510.400(a)(2). This measure is weighted at 40 percent of the composite quality score.

(3) Any additional quality improvement points the hospital may earn as a result of demonstrating improvement on either or both of the quality measures in paragraphs (b)(1) and (2) of this section, as described in paragraph (d) of this section.

(4) If applicable, 2 additional points for successful THA/TKA voluntary data submission of patient-reported outcomes and limited risk variable data, as described in §510.400(b). Successful submission is weighted at 10 percent of the composite quality score.

(c) *Quality performance points.* CMS computes quality performance points for each quality measure based on the participant hospital's performance percentile relative to the national distribution of all hospitals' performance on that measure.

(1) For the hospital-level risk-standardized complication rate following elective primary total hip arthroplasty and/or total knee arthroplasty measure (NQF #1550) described in §510.400(a)(1), CMS assigns the participant hospital measure value to a performance percentile and then quality performance points are

assigned based on the following performance l?ercentile scale:

(i) 10.00 pomts for 0th.
(ii) 9.25 points for 0th and <90th.
(iii) 8.50 points for <::70th and <80th;
(iv) 7.75 points for <::60th and <70th.
(v) 7.00 points for 50th and <60th.
(vi) 6.25 points for 40th and <50th.
(vii) 5.50 points for 0th and <40th.
(ix) 0.0 points for <30th.

(2) For the Hospital Consumer Assessment of Healthcare Providers and Systems Survey measure (NQF #0166) described in §510.400(a)(2), CMS assigns the participant hospital measure value to a performance percentile and quality performance points are assigned based on the following performance percentile scale;

(i) 8.00 points for 0th.
(ii) 7.40 points for 0th and <90th.
(iii) 6.80 points for 70th and <80th.
(iv) 6.20 points for <::60th and <70th.
(v) 5.60 points for 50th and <60th.
(vi) 5.00 points for 40th and <50th.
(vii) 4.40 points for 30th and <40th.
(ix) 0.0 points for <30th.

(d) *Quality improvement points.* !f a participant hospital's quality performance percentile on an individual measure described in §510.400(a) increases from the previous performance year by at least 3 deciles on the performance percentile scale, then the hospital is eligible to receive quality improvement points equal to 10 percent of the total available points for that individual measure.

(el *Exception for hospitals without a measure value.* Inthe case of a participant hospital without a measure value that would allow CMS to assign quality performance points for that quality measure, CMS assigns the 50th percentile quality performance points to the hospital for the individual measure.

(1) A participant hospital will not have a measure value for the-

(i) Hospital-level risk-standardized complication rate following elective primary total hip arthroplasty and/or total knee arthroplasty measure (NQF #1550) described in §510.400(a)(1) if the hospital does not meet the minimum 25 case count; or

(ii) Hospital Consumer Assessment of Healthcare Providers and Systems Survey measure (NQF #0166) described in §510.400(a)(2) if the hospital does not meet the minimum of 100 completed survey and does not have 4 consecutive quarters of HCAHPS data.

(ii) For either of the measures described in paragraphs (e)(1) or (2) of this section, if CMS identifies an error in the data used to calculate the measure and suppresses the measure value.

(t') *Quality incentive payments.* CMS provides incentive payments to

participant hospitals that demonstrate good or excellent quality performance on the composite quality scores described in paragraph (b) of this section. These incentive payments are implemented in the form of the following reductions to the applicable discount factors described in §510.300(c):

(1) A 1.0 percentage point reduction to the applicable discount factor for participant hospitals with good quality performance, defined as composite quality scores that are greater than or equal to 6.0 and less than or equal to 13.2.

(2) A 1.5 percentage point reduction to the applicable discount factor for participant hospitals with excellent quality performance, defined as composite quality scores that are greater than 13.2.

§510.320 Treatment of incentive programs or add-on payments under existing Medicare payment systems.

The CJR model does not replace any existing Medicare incentive programs or add-on payments. The target price and NPRA for a participant hospital are independent of, and do not affect, any incentive programs or add-on payments under existing Medicare payment systems.

§510.325 Allocation of payments tor services that straddle the episode.

(a) *General.* Services included in the episode that straddle the episode are prorated so that only the portion attributable to care furnished during the episode are included in the calculation of actual episode_payments.

(b) *Proration of seivices.* Payments for services that straddle the episode are prorated using the following methodology:

(1) *Non-IPPS inpatient selVices and other inpatient services.* Non-IPPS inpatient services, and services furnished by other inpatient providers that extend beyond the end of the episode are prorated according to the percentage of the actual length of stay (in days) that falls within the episode.

(2) *Home health agency sel'Vlces.* Home health services paid under the prospective payment system in part 484, subpart E of this chapter are prorated according to the percentage of days, starting with the first billable service date ("start of care date") and through and including the last billable service date, that occur during the episode. This methodology is applied in the same way if the home health services begin (the start of care date) prior to the start of the episode.

(3) *!PPS services.* IPPS claim amounts that extend beyond the end of the

episode are prorated according to the geometric mean length of stay, using the following methodology:

(i) The first day of the IPPS stay is counted as 2 days.

(ii) If the actual length of stay that occurred during the episode is equal to or greater than the MS-DRG geometric mean, the normal MS-DRG payment is fully allocated to the episode.

(iii) If the actual length of stay that occurred during the episode is less than the geometric mean, the normal MS-DRG payment amount is allocated to the episode based on the number of inpatient days that fall within the episode.

(iv) If the full amount is not allocated to the episode, any remainder amount is allocated to the post-episode spending calculation (defined in §510.2).

Subpart E--Quality Measures, Beneficiary Protections, and Compliance Enforcement

§510.400 Quality measures and reporting.

(a) *Reporting of quality measures.* The following quality measures are used for public reporting, for determining whether a participant hospital is eligible for reconciliation payments under §510.305(g), and whether a participant hospital is eligible for quality incentive payments under §510.315(f) in the performance year:

(1) Hospital-level risk-standardized complication rate following elective primary total hip arthroplasty and/or total knee arthroplasty.

(2) Hospital Consumer Assessment of Healthcare Providers and Systems Survey.

(b) *Requirements for successful voluntary data submission of patient-reported outcomes and limited risk variable data.* To be eligible to receive the additional points added to the composite quality score for successful voluntary data submission of patient-reported outcomes and limited risk variable data, as described in §510.315(b)(4), participant hospitals must submit the THA/TKA patient-reported outcome and limited risk variable data requested by CMS related to the pre- and post-operative periods for elective primary total hip and/or total knee arthroplasty procedures. The data must be submitted within 60 days of the end of the most recent performance period and be accompanied by the patient-reported outcomes and limited risk variable data (eleven elements finalized) as outlined in §510.315(b)(4).

(1) For each eligible procedure all eleven risk variable data elements are

required to be submitted. The eleven risk variables are as follows:

(i) Date of birth.
(ii) Race.
(iii) Ethnicity.
(iv) Date of admission to anchor hospitalization.
(v) Date of eligible THA/TKA procedure.
(vi) Medicare Health Insurance Claim Number.
(vii) Body mass index.
(viii) Use of chronic (>0 day) narcotics.
(ix) Total painful joint count.
(x) Quantified spinal pain.
(xi) Single Item Health Literacy Screening (SILS2) questionnaire.

(2) Hospitals must also submit the amount of requested THA/TKA patient-reported outcomes data required for each year of the model in order to be considered successful in submitting voluntary data.

(i) The amount of requested THA/TKA patient-reported outcomes data to submit, in order to be considered successful will increase each subsequent year of the model over the 5 years of the model.

(ii) A phase-in approach that determines the amount of requested THA/TKA patient-reported outcomes data to submit over the 5 years of the program will be applied so that in year 1 successful submission of data would mean CMS received all requested THA/TKA patient-reported outcomes and limited risk variable data on both of the following:

(A) Greater than or equal to 50 percent of eligible procedures or greater than or equal to 50 eligible patients during the data collection period.

(B) Submission of requested THA/TKA PRO and limited risk variable data is completed within 60 days of the most recent performance period.

(3) For years 1 through 5 of the model an increasing amount of data is requested by CMS for each performance period as follows:

(i) Year 1 (2016). Submit pre-operative data on primary elective THA/TKA procedures for <::50% or .:50 eligible procedures performed between July 1, 2016 and August 31, 2016, unless CMS requests a more limited data set, in which case, submit all requested data elements.

(ii) Year 2 (2017). Submit-
(A) Post-operative data on primary elective THA/TKA procedures for <::50% or .!:50 eligible procedures performed between July 1, 2016 through August 31, 2016; and

(B) Pre-operative data on primary elective THA/TKA procedures for ;,:so% or:.?:75 procedures performed

between September 1, 2016 through June 30, 2017, unless CMS requests a more limited data set, in which case, submit all requested data elements.

(iii) Year 3 (2018). Submit-
(A) POST-operative data on primary elective THA/TKA procedures for ::.?:SO% or ;,:75 procedures performed between September 1, 2016 and June 30, 2017; and

(B) Pre-operative data on primary elective THA/TKA procedures for <::70% or .!:100 procedures performed between July 1, 2017 and June 30, 2018, unless CMS requests a more limited data set, in which case, submit all requested data elements.

(iv) Year 4 (2019). Submit-
(A) Post-operative data on primary elective THA/TKA procedures for .!:70% or ;;;:100 procedures performed between July 1, 2017 and June 30, 2018; and

(B) Pre-operative data on primary elective THA/TKA procedures for ;;;:so% or ;;;:zoo procedures performed between July 1, 2018 and June 30, 2019, unless CMS requests a more limited data set, in which case, submit all requested data elements.

(v) Year 5 (2020). Submit-
(A) Post-operative data on primary elective THA/TKA procedures for ;;;:so% or ;;;:zoo procedures performed between July 1, 2018 and June 30, 2019 and

(B) Pre-operative data on primary elective THA/TKA procedures for ;;;:so% or ;;;:zoo procedures performed between July 1, 2019 and June 30, 2020, unless CMS requests a more limited data set, in which case, submit all requested data elements.

(c) *Public reporting.* CMS-
(1) Makes the quality measurement results calculated for the complication and patient survey quality measures described in paragraph (a) of this section for each participant hospital in each performance year publicly available on the CMS Web site in a form and manner as determined by CMS;

(2) Shares each participant hospital's quality metrics with the hospital prior to display on the Web site; and

(3) Does not publicly report the voluntary patient-reported outcomes and limited risk variable data during this model, but does indicate whether a hospital has voluntarily submitted such data.

§510.405 Beneficiary choice and beneficiary notification.

(a) *Beneficiary choice.* The CJR model does not restrict Medicare beneficiaries' ability to choose any Medicare enrolled provider or supplier, or any physician or practitioner who has opted out of Medicare.

51

(1) As part of discharge planning and referral, participant hospitals must inform beneficiaries of all Medicare participating post-acute care providers in an area and must identify those post-acute care providers with whom they have sharing arrangements. Participant hospitals may recommend preferred providers and suppliers, consistent with applicable statutes and regulations. Participant hospitals may not limit beneficiary choice to any list of providers or suppliers in any manner other than that permitted under applicable statutes and regulations. Participant hospitals must respect patient and family preferences when they are exl?ressed.

(2) Participant hospitals may not charge any CJR collaborator a fee to be included on any list of preferred providers or suppliers, nor may the participant hospital accept such payments.

(bl *Required beneficiary notification*-(1) *Hospital detailed notification.* Each participant hospital must provide written notice to any Medicare beneficiary that meets the criteria in §510.205 of his or her inclusion in the *CJR* model. The notice must be upon admission to the participant hospital or immediately following the decision to schedule an LEJR surgery, whichever occurs later. The beneficiary notification must contain all of the following:

(i) A detailed explanation of the model and how it might be expected to affect the beneficiary's care.

(ii) Notification that the beneficiary retains freedom of choice to choose providers and services.

(iii) Explanation of how patients can access care records and claims data through an available patient portal. and how they can share access to their Blue Button® electronic health information with caregivers.

(iv) A statement that all existing Medicare beneficiary protections continue to be available to the beneficiary. These include the ability to report concerns of substandard care to Quality Improvement Organizations and 1-800-MEDICARE.

(v) A list of the providers and suppliers with whom the participant hospital has a collaborator agreement.

(2) *Physician provision of notice.* A participant hospital must require any physician that is a CJR collaborator to provide written notice of the structure of the model and the existence of the physician's sharing arrangement with the participant hospital to any Medicare beneficiary that meets the criteria specified in §510.205. The notice must be provided at the time that the decision to undergo LE]R surgery is made.

(3) *PAC provider/supplier notification.* A participant hospital must require any provider or supplier, other than the treating physician discussed in paragraph (b)(2) of this section, with whom it has executed a collaborator agreement to provide written notice of the existence of its sharing arrangement with the participant hospital to any Medicare beneficiary that meets the criteria specified in §510.205. The notice must be provided no later than the time at which the beneficiary first receives services from the provider or supplier during the CJR episode.

[4] *Discharge planning notice.* A participant hospital must provide the beneficiary with a written notice of any potential financial liability, associated with non-covered services recommended or presented as an option as part of discharge planning, no later than the time that the beneficiary discusses a particular PAC option or at the time the beneficiary is discharged, whichever occurs earlier.

(i) If the hospital knows or should have known that the beneficiary is considering or has decided to receive a non-covered post-acute service or other non-covered associated service or supply, the hospital must notify the beneficiary that the service would not be covered by Medicare.

(ii) If the hospital is discharging a beneficiary to a SNF prior to the occurrence of a 3 day hospital stay, and the beneficiary is being transferred to or is considering a SNF that would not qualify under the SNF 3-day waiver in §510.610, the hospital notify the beneficiary in accordance with paragraph (b)(4)(i) of this section that the beneficiary will be responsible for costs associated with that stay except those which would be covered by Medicare Part B during a non-covered inpatient SNF stay.

§510.410 COmpllance enforcement

(a) *General.* Participant hospitals must comply with all of the requirements outlined in this part. Except as specifically noted in this part, the regulations under this part must not be construed to affect the payment, coverage, program integrity, or other requirements (such as those in parts 412 and 482 of this chapter) that apply to providers and suppliers under this chapter.

(l:i) *Failure to comply.* (1) CMS may take one or more of the remedial actions set forth in paragraph (b)(2) of this section if a participant hospital or any of the participant hospital's CJR collaborators-

(i) Fails to comply with any applicable requirements of this part or

is identified as noncompliant through monitoring by HHS (including CMS and OIG) of the CJR model, including but not limited to the following:

(A) Avoiding potentially high cost patients.

(Bl Targeting potentially low cost patients.

(Cl Failing to provide medically appropriate services or systematically engaging in the over or under delivery of appropriate care.

(DJ Failing to provide beneficiaries with complete and accurate information, including required notices.

(El Failing to allow beneficiary choice of medically necessary options, including non-surgical options.

(Fl Failing to follow the requirements related to collaborator agreements;

(ii) Has signed a collaborator agreement with a CJR collaborator if the agreement is noncompliant with the requirements of this part;

(iii) Takes any action that threatens the health or safety of patients;

(iv) Avoids at-risk Medicare beneficiaries, as this term is defined in §425.20;

(v) Avoids patients on the basis of payer status;

[vi) Is subject to sanctions or final actions of an accrediting organization or federal, state, or local government agency that could lead to the inability to comply with the requirements and provisions of this part;

(vii) Takes any action that CMS determines for program integrity reasons is not in the best interests of the CJR model, or fails to take any action that CMS determines for program integrity reasons should have been taken to further the best interests of the CJR model;

(viii) Is subject to action by HHS (including OIG and CMS) or the Department of Justice to redress an allegation of fraud or significant misconduct, including intervening in a False Claims Act qui tam matter, issuing a pre-demand or demand letter under a civil sanction authority, or similar actions; or

(ix) Is subject to action involving violations of the physician self-referral law, civil monetary penalties law, federal anti-kickback statute, antitrust laws, or any other applicable Medicare laws, rules, or regulations that are relevant to the CJR model.

(2) Remedial actions include the following:

(i) Issue a warning letter to the participant hospital.

(ii) Require tlie participant hospital to develop a corrective action plan, commonly referred to as a CAP.

(iii) Reduce or eliminate a participant hospital's reconciliation payment.

(iv) Require a participant hospital to terminate a collaborator agreement with a CJR collaborator and prohibit further engagement in the CJR model by that CJR collaborator.

(v) Terminate the participant hospital's participation in the CJR model.

(3) CMS may add 25 percent to a repayment amount on a participant hospital's reconciliation report if all of the following criteria are satisfied:

(i) CMS has required a corrective action plan from a participant hospital.

(ii) The participant hospital is not due a positive reconciliation payment but instead owes a repayment amount to CMS.

(iii) The participant hospital fails to timely comply with the corrective action plan or is noncompliant with the model's requirements.

Subpart F-Financial Arrangements and Beneficiary Incentives

§510.500 Financial arrangementa under the CJR model.

(al *General.* (1) A participant hospital may elect to enter into sharing arrangements.

(2) A participant hospital must not make a gainsharing payment or receive an alignment payment except in accordance with a sharing arrangement. Any gainsharing payments or alignment payments made in accordance with a sharing arrangement must be made only from the participant hospital to the CJR collaborator with whom the participant hospital has signed a collaborator agreement containing a sharing arrangement.

(3) CMS may review any sharing arrangement for compliance with the requirements of this part and to ensure that it does not pose a risk to beneficiary access, beneficiary freedom of choice, or quality of care.

(4) The participant hospital has ultimate responsibility for fully complying with all provisions of the CJR model.

(5) If a participant hospital enters into a sharing arrangement, it must update its compliance program to include oversight of sharing arrangements and compliance with the requirements of the CJR model.

(6) The board or other governing body of the participant hospital must have responsibility for overseeing the participant hospital's participation in the CJR model, its arrangements with CJR collaborators, its payment of gainsharing payments and receipt of alignment payments, and its use of beneficiary incentives in the CJR model.

(7) Participant hospitals must develop and maintain a written set of policies for selecting providers and suppliers for sharing gains and risk as CJR collaborators. This set of policies must contain criteria for selection of CJR collaborators related to, and inclusive of, the quality of care to be delivered by the CJR collaborator to beneficiaries during a CJR episode. The selection criteria cannot be based directly or indirectly on the volume or value of referrals or business otherwise generated by, between or among the participant hospital, CJR collaborators, and any individual or entity affiliated with a participant hospital or CJR collaborator. All collaborator agreements must require the CJR collaborator to have met, or agree to meet, the quality criteria for selection.

(b} *Sharing arrangement requirements.* Each sharing arrangement must comply with the following criteria:

(1) The sharing arrangement must be set forth in a collaborator agreement that complies with the requirements of paragraph (cl of this section.

(2) The sharing arrangement must comply with all relevant laws and regulations, including the applicable fraud and abuse laws and all applicable payi:nent and coverage requirements.

(3) An individual or entity's participation in a sharing arrangement must be voluntary and without penalty for nonparticipation.

(4) Tlie parties must enter into a sharing arrangement before care is furnished to CJR beneficiaries under the terms of the sharing arrangement.

(5)(i) To be eligible to receive a gainsharing payment, a CJR collaborator must meet quality criteria for the calendar year for which the gainsharing payment is determined by the participant hospital. The quality criteria must be established by the participant hospital and directly related to CJR episodes of care.

(ii) To be eligible to receive a gainsharing payment or make an alignment payment, a CJR collaborator other than a PCP must directly furnish a billable service to a CJR beneficiary during a CJR episode that occurred in the calendar year in which the savings or loss was created.

(iii) To be eligible to receive a gainsharing payment, a PCP that is a CJR collaborator must meet the following criteria:

(A) The PGP must have billed for an item or service that was rendered by one or more members of the PCP to a CJR beneficiary during a CJR episode that occurred during the calendar year in which the participant hospital's internal cost savings was generated, or to which the NPRA applied, the latter of which is contained in a reconciliation payment.

(Bl The PCP must contribute to a participant hospital's care redesign in the CJR model and be clinically involved in the care of CJR beneficiaries. The following is a non-exhaustive list of ways in which a PGP might be clinically involved in the care of CJR beneficiaries:

(1) Provide care coordination services to CJR beneficiaries during and/or after inpatient admission.

(2) Engage with a participant hospital in care redesign strategies, and actually perform a role in implementing such strategies, that are designed to improve the quality of care for LEJR episodes and reduce the LEJR episode spending.

(3) Incoordination with other providers and suppliers (such as members of the PGP, participant hospitals, post-acute care providers), implement strategies designed to address and manage the comorbidities of CJR beneficiaries.

(6) No entity or individual, whether a party to a collaborator agreement or not, may condition the opportunity to mak or receive gainsharing payments or to make or receive alignment payments on the volume or value of referrals or business otherwise generated by, between or among the participant hospital, CJR collaborators, and any individual or entity affiliated with a participant hospital or CJR collaborator.

(7) Gainsharing payments, if any, must be-

(i) Derived solely from reconciliation payments, or internal cost savings, or both;

(ii) Actually and proportionally related to the care of beneficiaries in a CJR episode;

(iii) Distributed on an annual basis (not more than once per calendar year);

(iv) Not be a loan, advance payments, or payments for referrals or other business; and

(v) Be clearly identified and comply with all provisions in this part, as well as all applicable laws, statutes, and rules.

(8) Alignment payments from a CJR collaborator to a participant hospital may be made at any interval that is agreed upon by both parties, and must-

(i) Not be issued, distributed, or paid prior to the calculation by CMS of a repayment amount reflected in a reconciliation report; and

(ii) Not be a loan, advance payments, or payments for referrals or other business.

(9) A participant hospital must not make a gainsharing payment to a CJR collaborator that is subject to any action for noncompliance with this part or the fraud and abuse laws, or for the

provision of substandard care in CJR episodes or other integrity problems.

(10) In a calendar year, the aggregate amount of all gainsharing payments distributed by a participant hospital that are derived from a CJR reconciliation payment may not exceed the amount of the reconciliation payment the participant hospital receives from CMS.

(11) In a calendar year, the aggregate amount of all alignment payments received by the participant hospital must not exceed 50 percent of the participant hospital's repayment amount No alignment payments may be collected by a participant hospital if it does not owe a repayment amount.

(12) The aggregate amount of all alignment payments from any one CJR collaborator to a participant hospital must not be greater than 25 percent of the participant hospital's repayment amount.

(13) A sharing arrangement must not induce the participant hospital, CJR collaborator, or any employees or contractors of the participant hospital or CJR collaborator to reduce or limit medically necessary services to any Medicare beneficiary.

(14) A sharing arrangement must not restrict the ability of a CJR collaborator to make decisions in the best interests of its patients, including the selection of devices, supplies, and treatments.

(15) The methodology for determining gainsharing payments must be based, at least in part, on criteria related to, and inclusive of, the quality of care to be delivered to CJR beneficiaries during an episode and must not directly account for the volume or value of referrals or business otherwise generated by, between or among the participant hospital. CJR collaborators, and any individual or entity affiliated with a participant hospital or CJR collaborator.

(16) The methodology for determining alignment payments must not directly account for the volume or value of referrals or business otherwise generated by, between or among the participant hospital. CJR collaborators, and any individual or entity affiliated with a participant hospital or CJR collaborator.

(17) The total amount of a gainsharing payment for a calendar year paid to an individual physician or nonphysician practitioner who is a CJR collaborator must not exceed 50 percent of the total Medicare approved amounts under the Physician Fee Schedule (PFS) for services furnished to the participant hospital's CJR beneficiaries during a CJR episode by that physician or nonphysician practitioner.

(18) The total amount of gainsharing payments for a calendar year paid to a

PGP that is a CJR collaborator must not exceed 50 percent of the total Medicare approved amounts under the Physician Fee Schedule for services that are billed by the PGP and furnished during a calendar year by members of the PGP to the participant hospital's CJR beneficiaries during CJR episodes.

(19) The participant hospital's determination of internal cost savings must satisfy the following criteria:

(i) Internal cost savings are calculated in accordance with generally accepted accounting principles and Government Auditing Standards (The Yellow Book).

(ii) All amounts determined to be internal cost savings must reflect actual, internal cost savings achieved by the participant hospital through implementation of care redesign elements identified and documented by the participant hospital. Internal cost savings does not include savings realized by any individual or entity that is not the participant hospital.

(iii) Internal cost savings may not reflect "paper" savings from accounting conventions or past investment in fixed costs.

(20) All gainsharing payments and any alignment payments must meet the requirements set forth in this section and be administered by the participant hospital in accordance with generally accepted accounting principles. In no event may the participant hospital receive any amounts from a CJR collaborator under a sharing arrangement that are not alignment payments.

(21) All gainsharing payments and alignment payments must be made through EFT.

(c) *Contents of collaborator agreement.* Each collaborator agreement must satisfy the following criteria:

(1) The collaborator agreement must contain a description of the sharing arrangement between the participant hospital and the CJR collaborator regarding gainsharing payments and alignment payments. This description must specify the following:

(i) The parties to the sharing arrangement.

(ii) The date of the sharing arrangement.

(iii) The purpose and scope of the sharing arrangement.

(iv) The financial or economic terms of the sharing arrangement, including the frequency of payment, and the methodology and accounting formula for determining the amount of any gainsharing payment or alignment payment

(v) Safeguards to ensure that alignment payments are made solely for purposes related to sharing

responsibility for funds needed to repay Medicare in the CJR model.

(vi) Plans regarding care redesign.

(vii) Changes in care coordination or delivery that is applied to the participant hospital or CJR collaborators or both.

(viii) A description of how success will be measured.

(ix) Management and staffing information, including type of personnel or contractors that will be primarily responsible for carrying out changes to care under the CJR model.

(2) The collaborator agreement must contain a requirement that the CJR collaborator and its employees and contractors must comply with the applicable provisions of this part (including requirements regarding beneficiary notifications, access to records, record retention, and participation in any evaluation, monitoring, compliance, and enforcement activities performed by CMS or its designees) and all other applicable laws and regulations.

(3) The collaborator agreement must require the CJR collaborator to be in compliance with all Medicare provider enrollment requirements at §424.500 of this chapter, including having a valid and active TIN or NPI, during the term of the agreement.

(4) The collaborator agreement must require the CJR collaborator to have a compliance program that includes oversight of the collaborator agreement and compliance with the requirements of the CJR model.

(5) The collaborator agreement must set forth a specific methodology for accruing, calculating, and verifying the internal cost savings generated by the participant hospital based on the care redesign elements specifically associated with the particular CJR collaborator.

(i) The methodology must set out the specific care redesign elements to be undertaken by the participant hospital or the CJR collaborator or both.

(ii) The methodology must be based, at least in part, on criteria related to, and inclusive of, the quality of care to be delivered to CJR beneficiaries during an episode and must not directly account for the volume or value of referrals or business otherwise generated by, between or among the participant hospital, CJR collaborators, and any individual or entity affiliated with a participant hospital or CJR collaborator.

(iii) The specific methodologies for accruing and calculating internal cost savings must be transparent, measurable, and verifiable in accordance with generally accepted accounting principles and Government Auditing Standards (The Yellow Book).

(6) The collaborator agreement must set forth the quality criteria established by the participant hospital that will be used in determining the gainsharing payment.

(7) The collaborator agreement must require the participant hospital to recoup gainsharing payments paid to CJR collaborators if gainsharing payments contain funds derived from a CMS overpayment on a reconciliation report, or were based on the submission of false or fraudulent data.

(d) *Documentation requirements.* (1) Documentation of any collaborator agreement containing a sharing arrangement must be contemporaneous with the establishment of the arrangement.

(2) A participant hospital must maintain accurate current and historical lists of all CJR collaborators, including names and addresses of each CJR collaborator. The participant hospital must update the lists on at least a quarterly basis and publicly report the current and historical lists of CJR collaborators on a public-facing Web page on the participant hospital's Web site.

(3) The participant hospital and CJR collaborator must maintain contemporaneous documentation of the payment or receipt of any gainsharing payment or alignment payment. The documentation must identify at least the following: The nature of the payment (gainsharing payment or alignment payment); the identity of the parties making and receiving the payment; the date of the payment; the amount of the payment; and the date and amount of any recoupment of all or a portion of a CJR collaborator's gainsharing payment.

(4) The participant hospital must keep records of the following:

(i) Its process for determining and verifying the eligibility of CJR collaborators to participate in Medicare.

(ii) Information confirming the organizational readiness of the participant hospital to measure and track internal cost savings.

(iii) The participant hospital's plan to track internal cost savings.

(iv) Information on the accounting systems used to track internal cost savings.

(v) A description of current health information technology, including systems to track reconciliation payments and internal cost savings.

(vi) The participant hospital's plan to track gainsharing payments and alignment payments.

(vii) Whether the participant hospital recouped any gainsharing payments

received by a CJR collaborator that contain funds derived from a CMS overpayment on a reconciliation report, or were based on the submission of false or fraudulent data.

(e) *Access to records and record retention.* All participant hospitals and CJR collaborators who enter into sharing arrangements must:

(1) Provide to CMS, the OIG, and the Comptroller General or their designees scheduled and unscheduled access to all books, contracts, records, documents, and other evidence (including data related to utilization and payments, quality criteria, billings, lists of CJR collaborators, sharing arrangements, and distribution arrangements, and the documentation required under paragraph (d) of this section) sufficient to enable the audit, evaluation, inspection, or investigation of the individual's or entity's compliance with CJR requirements, the quality of services furnished, the obligation to repay any reconciliation payments owed to CMS, or the calculation, distribution, receipt, or recoupment of gainsharing payments, alignment payments, or distribution payments.

(2) Maintain all such books, contracts, records, documents, and other evidence for a period of 10 years from the last day of the participant hospital's participation in the CJR model or from the date of completion of any audit, evaluation, inspection, or investigation, whichever is later, unless-

(i) CMS determines that there is a special need to retain a particular record or group of records for a longer period and notifies the participant hospital at least 30 calendar days before the normal disposition date; or

(ii) There has been a dispute or allegation of fraud or similar fault against the participant hospital or any CJR collaborator, in which case the records must be maintained for an additional 6 years from the date of any resulting final resolution of the dispute or allegation of fraud or similar fault.

§510.505 Distribution arrangements.

(a) *General.* (1) A PGP that has entered into a collaborator agreement with a participant hospital may distribute all or a portion of any gainsharing payment it receives from the hospital only in accordance with a distribution arrangement.

(2) All distribution arrangements must comply with the provisions of paragraph (b) of this section and all applicable laws and regulations, including the fraud and abuse laws.

(b) *Requirements.* (1) All distribution arrangements must be in writing and

signed by the PGP and practice collaboration ant.

(2) Participation in a distribution arrangement must be voluntary and without penalty for nonparticipation.

(3) The distribution arrangement must require the practice collaboration agent to comply with the requirements set forth in this part.

(4) The opportunity to receive a distribution payment must not be conditioned directly or indirectly on the volume or value of referrals or business otherwise generated by, between or among the participant hospital, PGP, other CJR collaborators, practice collaboration agents, and any individual or entity affiliated with a participant hospital, CJR collaborator, or practice collaboration agent.

(5) Methodologies for determining distribution payments must not directly account for volume or value of referrals, or business otherwise generated, by, between or among the participant hospital, PGP, other CJR collaborators, practice collaboration agents, and any individual or entity affiliated with a participant hospital, CJR collaborator, or practice collaboration agent.

(6) A practice collaboration agent is eligible to receive a distribution payment only if the PGP billed for an item or service furnished by the practice collaboration agent to a CJR beneficiary during a CJR episode that occurred during the calendar year in which the participating hospital accrued the internal cost savings or earned the reconciliation payment that comprise the gainsharing payment made to the PGP.

(7) When a PGP receives a gainsharing payment from a participant hospital in accordance with a sharing arrangement, all monies contained in such a gainsharing payment must be shared only with the physician or nonphysician practitioners that are PGP members that furnished a service to a CJR beneficiary during an episode of care in the calendar year from which the NPRA, as that term is defined in this part, or internal cost savings was generated, either or both of which are the only permitted sources of funds for a gainsharing payment.

(8) The total amount of distribution payments for a calendar year paid to a practice collaboration agent must not exceed 50 percent of the total Medicare approved amounts under the Physician Fee Schedule for services billed by the PGP and furnished by the practice collaboration agent to the participant hospital's CJR beneficiaries during a CJR episode.

(9) With respect to the distribution of any gainsharing payment received by a

PGP, the total amount of all distribution payments must not exceed the amount of the gainsharing payment.

(10) All distribution payments must be made through EFT.

(11) The practice collaboration agents must retain their ability to make decisions in the best interests of the patient, including the selection of devices, supplies, and treatments.

(12) The distribution arrangement must not-

(i) Induce a practice collaboration agent to reduce or limit medically necessary services to any Medicare beneficiary; or

(ii) Reward the provision of items and services that are medically unnecessary.

(13) The PGP must maintain contemporaneous documentation regarding distribution arrangements in accordance with §510.500(e), including the relevant written agreements, the date and amount of any distribution payment, the identity of each practice collaboration agent who received a distribution payment, and a description of the methodology and accounting formula for determining the amount of any distribution payment.

(14) The PGP may not enter into a distribution arrangement with any member of the PGP that has a collaborator agreement in effect with a participant hospital.

§510.510 Enforcement authority.

(a) *OIG authority.* OIG authority is not limited or restricted by the provisions of the CJR model, including the authority to audit, evaluate, investigate, or inspect the participant hospital, CJR collaborators, or any other person or entity or their records, data, or information, without limitation.

(b) *Other authorities.* None of the provisions of the CJR model limits or restricts the authority of any other government agency permitted by law to audit, evaluate, investigate, or inspect the participant hospital. CJR collaborators, or any other person or entity or their records, data, or information, without limitation.

§510.515 Bel18flclary IncentlVtlll under the CJR model.

(al *General.* Participant hospitals may choose to provide in-kind patient engagement incentives to beneficiaries in a CJR episode, subject to the following conditions:

(1) The incentive must be provided directly by the participant hospital or by an agent of the hospital under the hospital's direction and control to the beneficiary during a CJR episode of care.

(2) The item or service provided must be reasonably connected to medical care

provided to a beneficiary during an episode.

(3) The item or service must be a preventive care item or service or an item or service that advances a clinical goal, as listed in paragraph (bl of this section, for a beneficiary in a CJR episode by engaging the beneficiary in better managing his or her own health.

(4) The item or service must not be tied to the receipt of items or services outside the CJR episode of care.

(5) The item or service must not be tied to the receipt of items or services from a particular provider or supplier.

(6) The availability of the items or services must not be advertised or promoted except that a beneficiary may be made aware of the availability of the items or services at the time the beneficiary could reasonably benefit from them.

(7) The cost of the items or services must not be shifted to another federal health care program, as defined at section 1128B(f) of the Act.

(b) *Goals of the CJR model.* The following are the particular clinical goals of the CJR model. which may be advanced through beneficiary incentives:

(1) Beneficiary adherence to drug regimens.

(2) Beneficiary adherence to a care plan.

(3) Reduction of readmissions and complications resulting from LEJR procedures.

(4) Management of chronic diseases and conditions that may be affected by the lower extremity joint replacement procedure.

(cl *Documentation of beneficiary incentives.* (1) Participant hospitals must maintain documentation of items and services furnished as beneficiary incentives that exceed $25 in retail value.

(2) The documentation must be contemporaneous with the provision of the items and services and must include at least the following:

(i) The date the incentive is provided.

(ii) The identity of the beneficiary to whom the item or service was provided.

(3) The participant hospital must retain the required documentation in accordance with paragraph (el of this section.

(d) *Technology provided to a beneficiary.* (1) Items or services involving technology provided to a beneficiary may not exceed $1,000 in retail value for any one beneficiary in any one CJR episode.

(2) Items or services involving technology provided to a beneficiary must be the minimum necessary to advance a clinical goal, as listed in

paragraph (b) of this section, for a beneficiary in a CJR episode.

(3) Items of technology exceeding $100 in retail value must-

(i) Remain the property of the participant hospital; and

(ii) Be retrieved from the beneficiary at the end of the CJR episode. The participant hospital must document all retrieval attempts, including the ultimate date of retrieval. Documented, diligent, good faith attempts to retrieve items of technology will be deemed to meet the retrieval requirement.

(el *Documentation and maintenance of records.* All participant hospitals that provide in-kind patient engagement incentives to beneficiaries in CJR episodes must:

(1) Provide to CMS, the OIG, and the Comptroller General or their designee(s) scheduled and unscheduled access to all books, contracts, records, documents, and other evidence sufficient to enable the audit, evaluation, inspection, or investigation of the participant hospital's compliance with CJR requirements for beneficiary incentives.

(2) Maintain all such books, contracts, records, documents, and other evidence for a period of 10 years from the last day of the participant hospital's participation in the CJR model or from the date of completion of any audit, evaluation, inspection, or investigation, whichever is later, unless-

(i) CMS determines that there is a special need to retain a particular record or group of records for a longer period and notifies the participant hospital at least 30 calendar days before the normal disv.osition rate; or

(ii) There has been a dispute or allegation of fraud or similar fault against the participant hospital, in which case the records must be maintained for an additional 6 years from the date of any resulting final resolution of the dispute or allegation of fraud or similar fault.

Subpart G-Waivers

§510.600 Waiver of direct supervision requirement for certain postlacharge home visits.

(a) *General.* CMS waives the requirement in §410.26(b)(5) of this chapter that services and supplies furnished incident to a physician's service must be furnished under the direct supervision of the physician (or other practitioner) to permit home visits as specified in this section. The services furnished under this waiver are not considered to be "hospital services," even when furnished by the clinical staff of the hospital.

(b) *General supervision of qualified personnel.* The waiver of the direct supervision requirement in §410.26(b)(5) of this chapter applies only in the following circumstances:

(1) The home visit is furnished during the episode to a beneficiary who has been discharged from an anchor hospitalization.

(2) The home visit is furnished at the beneficiary's home or place of residence.

(3l The beneficiary does not qualify for home health services under sections 1835(al and 1814(al of the Act at the time of any such home visit.

(4l The visit is furnished by clinical staff under the general supervision of a physician or non-physician practitioner. Clinical staff are individuals who work under the supervision of a physician or other qualified health care professional, and who are allowed by law, regulation, and facility policy to perform or assist in the performance of a specific professional service, but do not individually report that professional service.

(5l No more than 9 visits are furnished to the beneficiary during the episode.

(cl *Payment.* Up to 9 post-discharge home visits per CJR episode may be billed under Part B by the physician or nonphysician practitioner or by the participant hospital to which the supervising physician has reassigned his or her billing rights.

(dl *Other requirements.* All other Medicare rules for coverage and payment of services incident to a physician's service continue to apply.

§510.605 Waiver of certain telehealth requirements.

(al *Waiver of the geographic site requirements.* Except for the geographic site requirements for a face-to-face encounter for home health certification, CMS waives the geographic site requirements of section 1834(ml(4l(C}(i}(I) through (ill} of the Act for episodes being tested in the CJR model, but only for services that—

(1) May be furnished via telehealth under existing requirements; and

(2) Are included in the episode in accordance with §510.200(bl.

(bl *Waiver of the originating site requirements.* Except for the originating site requirements for a face-to-face encounter for home health certification, CMS waives the originating site requirements under section 1834(m)(4)(C)(ii)(Il through (VlIl) of the Act for episodes being tested in the CJR model to permit a telehealth visit to originate in the beneficiary's home or place of residence, but only for services that—

(1} May be furnished via telehealth under existing requirements; and

(2l Are included in the CJR episode in accordance with §510.200(b).

(c) *Waiver of selected payment provisions.* (tl CMS waives the payment requirements under section 1834(m)(2)(A) so that the facility fee normally paid by Medicare to an originating site for a telehealth service is not paid if the service is originated in the beneficiary's home or place of residence.

(2) CMS waives the payment requirements under section 1834(m}(2)(B) to allow the distant site payment for telehealth home visit HCPCS codes unique to this model to more accurately reflect the resources involved in furnishing these services in the home by basing payment upon the comparable office visit relative value units for work and malpractice under the Physician Fee Schedule.

(d) *Other requirements.* All other requirements for Medicare coverage and payment of telehealth services continue to apply, including the list of specific services approved to be furnished by telehealth.

§510.610 Waiver of SNF 3-day rule.

(al *Waiver of the SNF 3-day rule.* For episodes being tested in the CJR model in performance years 2 through 5, CMS waives the SNF 3-day rule for coverage of a SNF stay for a CJR beneficiary following the anchor hospitalization, but only if the SNF is identified on the applicable calendar quarter list of qualified SNFs at the time of CJR beneficiary admission to the SNF.

(1) CMS determines the qualified SNFs for each calendar quarter based on a review of the most recent rolling 12 months of overall star ratings on the Five-Star Quality Rating System for SNFs on the Nursing Home Compare Web site. Qualified SNFs are rated an overall of 3 stars or better for at least 7 of the 12 months.

(2l CMS posts to the CMS Web site the list of qualified SNFs in advance of the calendar quarter and the waiver only applies for a beneficiary who has been discharged from an anchor hospitalization if the SNF is included on the applicable calendar quarter list for the date of the beneficiary's admission to the SNF.

(b) *Other requirements.* All other Medicare rules for coverage and payment of Part A-covered SNF services continue to apply.

§510.615 Waiver of certain poat-operative billing restrictions.

(al *Waiver to permit certain services to be billed separately during the 90-day post-operative global surgical period.* CMS waives the billing requirements for global surgeries to allow the separate billing of certain post-discharge home visits described under §510.600, including those related to recovery from the surgery, as described in paragraph (b} of this section, for episodes being tested in the CJR model.

(bl *Services to which the waiver applies.* Up to 9 post-discharge home visits, including those related to recovery from the surgery, per CJR episode may be billed separately under Part B by the physician or nonphysician practitioner, or by the participant hospital to which the physician or nonphysician practitioner has reassigned his or her billing rights.

(cl *Other requirements.* All other Medicare rules for global surgery billing during the 90-day post-operative period continue to apply.

§510.620 Waiver of deductible and coinsurance that otherwiee apply to reconciliation payments or repayments.

(al *Waiver af deductible and coinsurance.* CMS waives the requirements of sections 1813 and 1822(a) of the Act for Medicare Part A and Part B payment systems only to the extent necessary to make reconciliation payments or receive repayments based on the NPRA that reflect the episode payment methodology under the final payment model for CJR participant hospitals.

(ti) *Reconciliation payments or repayments.* Reconciliation payments or repayments do not affect the beneficiary cost-sharing amounts for the Part A and Part B services provided under the CJR model.

Subparts H–J [Reserved]

Subpart K—Model Termination

§510.900. Tennlnation of the CJR model.

CMS may terminate the CJR model for reasons including but not limited to the following:

(a) CMS determines that it no longer bas the funds to support the CJR model.

(b) CMS terminates the model in accordance with section 1115A(b)(3)(B) of the Act. As provided by section 1115A(d)(2} of the Act, termination of the model is not subject to administrative or judicial review.

Dated: November 2, 2015.

Andrew M. Slavitt,

Acting Administrator, Centers for Medicare & Medicaid Services.

Dated: November 9, 2015.

Sylvia M. Burwell,

Secretary, Department of Health and Human Services.

[FR Doc. 2015-29438 Filed 11-16-15; 4:15 pm]

BILI.ING CODE 4 1 –...P